Immunology:

The Many-Edged Sword

Immunology:

The Many-Edged Sword

HAROLD M. SCHMECK, JR.

GEORGE BRAZILLER

NEW YORK

To Peter

FOREWORD

The immune response is a natural phenomenon of disease that has long been recognized. Very early in recorded history references were made to the fact that recovery from a current "plague" protected a person against a second attack.

In the late eighteenth century, physicians began to find ways to mimic this naturally acquired immunity. Jenner developed a vaccine against smallpox and since then, one by one, infectious diseases have been yielding to the march of science.

It was not until early in this century, however, that immunology was established as a scientific discipline. As the major components of the immune response—antigens, antibodies, specialized cells, and complement—were identified, the amazingly complex manner in which the body protects itself against foreign invaders was revealed.

Scientists engaged in opening the new field of immunology have had their share of Nobel Prizes, beginning with Von Behring in 1901 who was honored for his work on the serum treatment of diphtheria. In 1908 a German, Ehrlich, and a Russian, Metchnikoff, were recognized for their work on immunity and in 1913, Richet's study of the overwhelming immune reaction known as anaphylaxis was similarly honored. Other Nobel Prize winners whose field was immunology include Bordet, Landsteiner, Burnet, Medawar, Edelman, and Porter. The last two shared the 1972 Prize for their separate research on the chemical structure of antibodies.

Since World War II, vigorous federal support of training and research—in which the National Institutes of Health has played a major role—has opened up new areas of immunology. The number of scientists engaged in research in this field has been rapidly increasing, as is shown by the burgeoning membership list of the American Association of Immunologists. This professional society has grown from less than 500 in the 1950s to over 1,200 in the 1970s. In addition, at many universities, immunologists have been appointed chairmen of principal departments such as pathology, microbiology, and medicine and provide expert leadership in research and teaching.

The volume of material published by immunologists has trebled in the last 15 years. New journals have sprung up and textbooks written. Immunologists have met in conferences and workshops and their discussions have formed the basis for numerous books of a highly technical nature.

But this explosion of scientific literature has not been matched by an increase in the number of books or articles on immunology suitable for the layman. Like most professionals, immunologists find themselves talking mostly to each other, and using a jargon not always understood even by other scientists.

In an attempt to break down this semantic wall, the National Institute of Allergy and Infectious Diseases, over the last six years, has sponsored several science writers' seminars and briefings in which Harold Schmeck has participated. In addition, Mr. Schmeck has established a close rapport with many of our scientists at the National Institutes of Health and with NIH grantees across the country. This long association makes it a special pleasure to welcome his book to that rather small body of literature that brings to the attention of all interested readers the exciting findings and continuing challenge of research in immunology.

DORLAND J. DAVIS, M.D.
Director, National Institute of Allergy and Infectious Diseases, National Institutes of Health.

CONTENTS

PREFACE

Immunology is a subject close to the essence of life and also full of immediate practical implications for human health. It is as prosaic as a smallpox vaccination or the runny nose that goes with the common cold. It is almost as mysterious as the first emergence of life in our planet's early seas.

Indeed, some features of the immunological defenses probably arose as a recognition system allowing primordial living things to solve the world's first identity crisis. To survive they had to possess means of distinguishing their own special chemical compounds and molecular structures from the rest of the dilute soup of organic chemicals on which they fed and whence they came.

Today, features of that recognition system that must have evolved from life's early experiments tell one type of blood from another, identify and guard against newly-formed cancer cells and perform other functions. Some of these, presumably, are yet to be discovered. It is the immunological defense system that protects against germs through vaccines and natural immunity and does many other things, some good, some bad.

The same basic system that produces immunity also produces common allergy and more serious kinds of self-inflicted illness.

The thrust of immunological research today is to make the defense system work harder in preventing and curing disease; and also, paradoxically, to make it less vigorous when its vigor is harmful to health. Some medical scientists seek ways to make the cancer patient's immune system fight harder against a tumor. Others seek a contrived truce between a transplanted kidney and the normal immune defenses that would destroy it. The two lines of research are simply opposite faces of the same coin. A project aimed at one objective often helps attain the other.

Immune processes are fundamental to the economy of life for all of earth's most complex living creatures. The hallmark of these processes is their exquisite gift for discrimination. The immune system can readily tell apart two virus particles so small that they can be seen only under the electron microscope and so closely related that they appear identical even in that view. For all these reasons immunology has become a universal tool in medical research.

Because the great defense system seems so widely involved in issues of health and illness, the subject is scientifically fashionable right now. Immunology seems to hold great promise for dealing with many of the most difficult problems of human disease. Cancer is one prime example. Arthritis is another.

But most of the promise of immunological warfare

against these major diseases is yet to be realized. The realization depends on further research. Scientists probe the interlocking puzzles of immunity out of curiosity and wonder, and also for reasons that are intensely practical. To the public and the government, the practical goals are urgent. The curiosity-for-its-own-sake may seem a dispensable luxury, but this is a dangerous illusion. The two aspects of scientific work are inseparable. A straight line is not always the shortest distance to victory over disease. The key to the practical end is often a chance discovery made by someone looking in another direction.

The purpose of this book is to give the reader a glimpse of what is going on in immunological research today and some appreciation of what it all means and why it is ultimately so important. The origin of the book was a series of four articles published in *The New York Times* in 1972. These have been expanded and revised to constitute chapters 2, 3, 4, and 6. I am deeply indebted to *The Times* for allowing me to use here the material from the four original articles and for encouraging me to write about developments in immunology during the past several years.

I would also like to express appreciation to the many scientists who have given me their time and help during those years. This book and the articles from which it developed would have been impossible without their generous help.

Below is a list of some of those to whom I am most indebted for guidance in the frontier world of immunology. To the extent that I have been able to glimpse the breathtaking vistas of that world, the credit is largely theirs. If I have stumbled into any quicksands of error on the journey, the fault is entirely mine.

D. Bernard Amos, K. Frank Austen, Fritz H. Bach, John J. Bergan, Mortimer M. Bortin, Charles G. Cochrane, Melvin Cohn, John R. David, Richard W. Dutton, Gerald M. Edelman, John L. Fahey, Clarence J. Gibbs, Jr., Robert A. Good, John G. Gorman, Michael Hanna, Karl Erik and Igegerd Hellstrom, Kimishige Ishizaka, Donald E. Kayhoe, Edmund Klein, Samuel L. Kountz, Maurice Landy, H. Sherwood Lawrence, E. Bruce Merchant, Donald L. Morton, Hugh O. McDevitt, Hans J. Muller-Eberhard, William E. Paul, Felix T. Rapaport, Frank J. Rauscher, Jr., Herbert J. Rapp, Paul Russell, Hilliard F. Seigler, Richard L. Simmons, Hans Olov Sjogren, Richard T. Smith, George Santos, Norman Shumway, William D. Terry, Paul I. Terasaki, E. Donnall Thomas.

H.M.S., JR.

1

IMMUNOLOGY,
BUTTERFLIES,
AND BLOOD

T

HEY were one of those young couples for whom the world seemed to be made—happy, healthy, intelligent, and full of enthusiasm for life. Their first baby was just like them. Anyone could see that a wonderful new family was coming into being.

But their next baby died soon after birth and the one after that was stillborn. They lost the next one, too, and the one after that. They finally gave up after multiple tragedies that left a mark on their lives.

There was nothing at all wrong with the health of either parent. In a sense they were victims of a statistical accident. Their problem was simply that the wife had Rh negative blood and the father was Rh positive.

Their first baby was Rh positive also and a few of its red blood cells escaped into the mother's circulation and sensitized her against blood of that type.

By the time of her next pregnancy with another baby of the same blood type, the mother's internal defense system was primed to destroy Rh positive blood cells. The result was fatal anemia in the baby. Long before doctors had any idea what caused this they gave it a name—*erythroblastosis fetalis.*

It used to cause the deaths of about 3,000 American babies a year and severe illness, often with permanent brain damage, in about seven times that many.

But new cases have become a rarity in this country since about 1968 because doctors found out, first, what caused it and, later, how it could be prevented. The story is one of the triumphs of modern immunology—the branch of science that deals with antibodies and immunity and all the complex factors in the body's system of internal self-defense.

Before the 1940s *erythroblastosis fetalis* was considered an inherited disease. A standard reference work said it was "due to an abnormal proportion of colorless cells from bone marrow in the blood which usurp the place of the erythrocytes."

Erythrocytes are red blood cells. The doctors who phrased that description of the disease had really observed the destructive effects of the mother's sensitized blood on the baby's red blood cells, but they didn't realize it.

The Rh factor itself wasn't discovered until about 1940. Shortly after that, Rh incompatibility between mother and infant was found to be at the root of the problem. Those key discoveries made it possible to save some of the threatened babies by exchange transfusions—replacement of all of the baby's blood soon after birth. More recently, early induced births and even transfusions while the baby was still in the womb have been tried in efforts to give some of these infants a better chance.

But these were all heroic measures taken in the face of

disaster after the deadly antagonism between the two blood streams had begun to work. These remedies weren't always successful and they did nothing at all to solve the basic problem. The mother who faced the harrowing crisis of Rh disease with her second baby could look forward to the probability that it would happen again and again. It was a cruel trick of fate engineered by nothing more nor less than the chance occurrence that she was one of the minority who have Rh negative blood while her husband was among the Rh positive majority.

Furthermore, once sensitized, the woman would stay that way forever.

A brighter outlook for Rh negative mothers began to form at about the beginning of the 1960s because medical scientists in two countries, specializing in several disciplines, were all drawn toward the problem by their own special interests.

In a way it is a classic case because it includes many of the features scientists like to point to as examples of the way progress is made. For one thing, the key discoveries were made almost simultaneously, and quite independently of each other, in England and the United States. A second point was that all the participants were more or less amateurs in this particular field. When they got the new idea that ultimately solved the problem, the established professionals in *erythroblastosis fetalis* would have none of it.

One of the Americans involved in the effort recalls that they were turned down twice by the National Institutes of Health when they applied for a research grant.

21

A third classic feature of the story was that the new scientific advance was built on a massive background of knowledge. There were important new discoveries, but there were also some observations that dated back to about 1909. Furthermore, some of the key ingredients to the ultimate success came from fields that had nothing to do with health problems of the newborn.

Among the scientists who became involved in the problem were two young doctors in New York—one an obstetrician, the other a pathologist with a particular interest in blood banking. They were joined by an immunologist who worked for a drug firm in New Jersey. Independently of them, a British team was also forming, led by a prominent geneticist who had a particular interest in butterflies.

On both sides of the Atlantic, the research benefited greatly from something that was developed in Germany about 1958. This was a highly sensitive test to show the presence of fetal blood cells in the mother's blood.

After several years of research, the American and British teams came independently to the same conclusions and arrived at the same solution almost at the same time. Then they found that a doctor in St. Louis had by-passed many of the steps they took and had proved the point at least as soon as they did.

Two of the key men on the team that organized itself in New York were at Columbia Presbyterian Medical Center. The obstetrician was Dr. Vincent J. Freda, who had recently finished his residency. He had already decided to commit

22

part of his career to an assault on *erythroblastosis fetalis.*

The pathologist was Dr. John G. Gorman, who was assistant director of the medical center's blood bank. He, too, had just completed a residency and was interested both in blood diseases and some of the central puzzles of immunology.

Dr. Freda enlisted Dr. Gorman's interest. This was easy to do partly because the Rh disease was a problem in which both diagnosis and treatment depended on the special resources of blood banks.

The two doctors started by studying the medical center's records of every mother who had experienced the blood problem there since 1946. Through these records one could watch the tide of anti-Rh antibodies ebb and flow in several generations of patients. The appearance of the antibodies matched fatefully with the damage to the babies.

The third man who joined the team was Dr. William Pollack, an immunologist and blood fraction expert on the staff of Ortho Pharmaceutical Corporation in New Jersey. In 1960 he came to Columbia to give a lecture on a blood test used to identify Rh negative persons. The three doctors talked after the lecture and, from that conversation, joined forces for a cooperative effort.

They knew that the key to the disease was the sensitization of the mother against Rh positive blood, a point proven years earlier by Dr. Philip Levine of New Jersey. They also knew from Dr. Levine's work that the Rh negative woman would have no problem unless she did become sensitized to the Rh factor. It is for that reason that such a

23

woman seldom has difficulty with her first pregnancy. She hasn't yet been sensitized.

So the question was: how to prevent that sensitization?

What turned out to be the real answer had been noticed as early as 1909 by the famous American pathologist Dr. Theobald Smith. To him it was an irksome, but inescapable fact that was barring the way to a successful vaccine against diphtheria. The logical way of preventing this dread disease was to give each person a mixture of diphtheria toxin (the poison) and antitoxin (the antibodies that protected against it). The objective was to produce immunity, but to do so without any danger of producing the disease.

It didn't work. One of the reasons, as Dr. Smith noted, was that the presence of the antitoxin prevented the development of permanent immunity.

In his study of the Rh problem in the early 1960s, Dr. Gorman recalls, it became clear that this phenomenon had been discovered over and over again. It hampered work against diphtheria in the early 1900s. It plagued research workers involved with tetanus in the 1920s; and then whooping cough and, still later, polio.

The common finding was this: if you give a person someone else's antibodies to protect against something dangerous, you may achieve the protection as long as those antibodies last—but no longer. The borrowed antibodies actually prevent development of lasting immunity against their own special target.

Each time the phenomenon appeared and thwarted a

vaccine development effort, scientists noted it with displeasure and then found a way to circumvent it. Hardly anyone seemed to notice it as an important biological principle.

A few medical scientists did notice. Among them were Drs. Gareth Gladstone and Edward P. Abraham. They contributed a chapter to W.B. Saunders Company's textbook on General Pathology edited by Dr. Howard Florey who had gained fame as a contributor to the development of penicillin. In their chapter they noted and described this effect of passive immunity (the injection of borrowed antibodies) in preventing a person from developing natural active immunity against the same target.

Perhaps it was a natural feedback effect—the body, sensing somehow that it had enough antibodies to deal with the problem at hand, signaled its antibody factories to stop making more. But, since these antibodies were borrowed, the person who received them had not yet made any. So the shutdown order would prevent the start of the very process the doctors were trying to trigger.

Whether or not that explanation is correct, the phenomenon was just the kind of clue the team in New York needed in the early 1960s. Active immunity to Rh positive blood was just exactly what they wanted to prevent.

While the doctors who were worrying about Rh disease spoke of sensitization and those trying to prevent diphtheria, tetanus, or polio spoke of immunization, they all meant the same thing. It has always been customary to use the word "immunity" when the effect is considered desirable, and "sensitization" when it is something to be avoided. Biologically the two are the same.

Whichever term was used to describe the phenomenon, the very effect that had been a serious hindrance to the earlier scientists began to look like the road to salvation to the men working against Rh disease.

Meanwhile, in England, a group at the University of Liverpool was coming to the same conclusion by a somewhat different route.

Two of the most important figures in the research in England were Dr. Ronald Finn and Dr. C. A. Clarke. Dr. Finn was a young medical scientist who took on the Rh problem as an assigned research project, although he had no background in that special field. Dr. Clarke was a prominent medical geneticist. Among other things, Dr. Clarke had a long standing interest in butterflies. During the 1950s he had studied the genetic patterns controlling the wing-colors in some species. He noticed certain striking parallels between a butterfly's inheritance of wing patterns and the inheritance of blood groups in man. The important point, so far as the Rh problem was concerned, was that because of the genetics of the situation other blood groups could interfere with a person's production of antibodies against the Rh factor.

This had been noticed years earlier by Dr. Levine in the U.S., who had found that a woman who had a strong ABO blood group incompatibility with her husband seldom had the Rh problem even if she was Rh negative. The logical explanation seemed to be that her preformed antibodies against the major blood group, whether it be A or B, would attack any foreign blood cells, including those that were Rh positive, before she had a chance to become sensitized to the Rh factor itself.

On both sides of the Atlantic, the solution finally appeared clear: give the mother antibodies against Rh positive blood soon after the birth of her first Rh positive child. These borrowed antibodies would sop up any blood cells from the baby that had escaped into the mother's circulation and prevent them from sensitizing the mother.

Dr. Clarke has said his wife woke him up in the middle of the night to tell him she thought anti-Rh antibodies were the answer; and he went back to sleep in a grouch because the idea at first seemed preposterous. After all, these antibodies were just what they were trying to prevent.

He soon realized that the strategy was correct; just as Drs. Gorman, Freda, and Pollack did after musing on the problems Theobald Smith had encountered with diphtheria vaccine more than fifty years previously.

It took a lot more research and testing to translate the basic idea to a practical form of routine treatment, but things that had to be done and the ways of doing them seemed to fall into place logically after that.

First the idea had to be tested in male volunteers. This was necessary to prove that the antibody injections would prevent sensitization against Rh positive blood and would not, by some unforeseen change, actually sensitize. It

27

seemed safer to do these first tests in men. If they were accidentally sensitized against the foreign blood type it would wasn't likely to do them any harm. If the first tests had been done in women—and had turned out badly—the women would be at risk of the Rh baby problem for the rest of their lives.

On both sides of the Atlantic both studies turned out the way the doctors had hoped they would. The next and final step was to try the method with Rh negative mothers who had just given birth to their first babies. That worked too and proved the point. The conquest of the Rh baby problem was at hand.

About that time, at a scientific meeting, Dr. Gorman was introduced to Dr. Eugene Hamilton of St. Louis who had proved the same point singlehandedly himself. When the doctors in New York were just getting their conclusions nailed down, Dr. Gorman recalls, Dr. Hamilton had amassed enough experience to equal the total of what everyone else had done all over the world.

There had been some theoretical discussion of the Rh problem in the early 1960s. In fact, Dr. Clarke had set forth the whole basis for the prevention of Rh disease in an article in the British Medical Journal. It wasn't based on actual experience. The studies in New York and Liverpool were yet to be done, but it did spell out the theory and suggested the practical steps that would have to be taken.

Dr. Gorman believes the influence of that article was profound and beneficial. Dr. Clarke's prominence gave the idea respectability among the "professionals" of *erythro-*

blastosis fetalis for the first time and, in fact, made it easier to get research support.

In St. Louis, Dr. Hamilton, reasoning that gamma globulin had been used for years for other purposes and was safe, tried the idea on some of his patients and it worked. By the time Dr. Gorman met him, Dr. Hamilton had more practical experience on patients with the revolutionary new method than anyone else.

The tragedies that occurred before 1968 seem almost needless now, but that is a judgment of hindsight. In earlier years these dead and damaged babies had to be viewed fatalistically as part of the inevitable toll of nature's mistakes. It took scientists who were willing to question the inevitable to see the situation otherwise.

Even so, the story doesn't quite live up to the fairy tale finale of "they all lived happily ever after."

Dr. Gorman said licensing of the gamma globulin product that has answered the problem was delayed several years in the 1960s for reasons that he considers tragically picayune.

He said licensing of the product was delayed by officials of the federal agency responsible for vaccines and other biologics products because they were worried about possible adverse side effects. These officials of the Division of Biologics Standards of the National Institutes of Health held up licensure until they were completely satisfied.

So, in Dr. Gorman's view, use of the drug that has been saving lives ever since, was seriously delayed because of fears that it might also cause a few skin rashes.

Furthermore, even today in the United States, it appears

that some women who should be treated are being overlooked and therefore must face the fear of the Rh disease
in their babies for the rest of their child-bearing years. In
particular, women who have abortions are being overlooked
when they too should be tested to see whether or not they
need the anti-Rh treatment.

There are some inevitable failures, because there are a
few women in whom the preventive measure doesn't seem
to work. But, altogether, about 20 percent of American
mothers who do need the treatment, are not getting it, according to current estimates. The score in Britain about
equals ours, but some other countries including Canada,
Australia, and the Netherlands are doing a substantially
better job. There are some other countries, even in Europe,
where usage of the preventive method is low—partly because of the expense.

Nevertheless, the defeat of *erythroblastosis fetalis* is a
classic international success story of medical science, a
story of imagination, persistence and courage that have
saved many lives. Immunologists tend to point to it with
particular pride because every aspect of the cause, understanding, and ultimate prevention of the disease rests on
one or another feature of that realm of science. What was
necessary was for the diverse students of immunology, butterflies, and blood to put it all together.

2

THE INVISIBLE
HOST

I

NSIDE the human body cells talk to one another continually in a conversation that makes the difference between health and illness, life and death. It is a dialogue that has been going on in a multitude of animal species probably for more than 300 million years. Its language is something that modern scientists call immunology.

Today, as the fund of knowledge seems to be mushrooming virtually month by month, specialists have a sense of real excitement. The incredibly complex system of immunology is yielding up a detailed understanding of what it really is and how it works.

Some scientists expect that their understanding will recast much of what medicine can do about many of man's most important diseases, including cancer, arthritis, and some forms of heart and kidney disease. Most of this promise is still to be realized; it is little more than a gleam in scientists' eyes.

Yet new ways to help the sick by manipulating the immunological system, unimaginable a few years ago, are already being tried. In technical reports, speeches, and informal conversations, scientists from many laboratories have made it clear that they have far more ambitious ideas for the future.

To support research in immunology, the National Institutes of Health (known collectively as the NIH) are spending about $64 million a year through grants and contracts, with most of it administered through the National Institute of Allergy and Infectious Diseases and the National Cancer Institute.

During the past two decades, the allergy and infectious diseases institute of the NIH has been the main source of research support and training in the field of immunology in the United States. In 1972 this institute organized a special task force of experts to assess the current "state of the art" in their rapidly developing field.

The assignment was to summarize current knowledge of the role of immunologic processes in health and illness and the importance of this knowledge in actual medical practice. The objective was to speed the discovery of important new knowledge and its translation into things useful to human health. A first draft of the task force report was completed by the end of 1972, with final publication planned for the following year.

That project was one of several recent efforts to focus specialists' attention on immunology in ways calculated to speed the pace of scientific progress and hasten the translation of science into medical practice and public health policy.

There are already several unconventional ways in which doctors are now manipulating the immune response to cope with disease.

One is the transplantation of bone marrow to give a

patient vital elements of a new and functional immunological system. Another is the use of a rather mysterious substance called "transfer factor" to give patients with defective immunological systems the capability to fight deadly infections against which they had been helpless. Both methods have already saved lives, although the illnesses against which they have been used are rare.

There are even more new manipulations that are still in the laboratory or animal research stage but that seem likely to be applied before long to human needs. Among them are such ideas as that of selectively removing particular harmful antibodies from the blood or preparing tailor-made magic bullets that would seek out and kill certain specific cells and no others in the body.

In these cases it is not so much the ideas that are new as the specificity with which the job can now be done. It is the difference between the bludgeon and the rapier, the blunderbuss and the rifle.

In the preface to the proceedings of the fourth in an annual series of conferences on immunology, Dr. Maurice Landy, of the National Institute of Allergy and Infectious Diseases, and Dr. Jonathan W. Uhr, then of New York University, said of the state of their art:

"The precision and selectivity of the forms of intervention envisioned for the immediate future will assuredly have an immense impact on medicine."

While immunology is one of the newest frontiers of medical science, it is also one of the oldest allies of medical practice. Doctors were making good use of it centuries before they had any real idea of what it was, or had even given it a name.

Today the most common use of immunology by far is vaccination, which got its scientific start in 1796 when Dr. Edward Jenner infected an eight-year-old boy with cowpox virus (vaccinia) in the hope that it would protect against smallpox.

Jenner's experiment gave us the very word "vaccination" —the agent of cowpox is called vaccinia virus after the Latin for cow—and freedom from one of the most dread and devastating diseases of man.

In modern terms, the fact that it did work would be explained by saying that the vaccination prevented the infectious disease by giving the body an immunologic memory of a virus that it had never met in the natural course of things. The agents of that memory are called antibodies.

Most nonscientists who ever think about it see the immunologic system simply as a defense against infection—a matter of antibodies made by the body to kill germs.

To a specialist the system now appears to comprise at least three kinds of living cells and five kinds of antibodies as well as other substances in a multitude of complex relationships that have an amazing range of vital functions.

It is clearly a main defense against infection. It appears to maintain surveillance continually against cancer. It maintains body integrity in important ways by distinguishing between "self" and "nonself" and, for that reason, it probably played an important role in evolution.

When the first living things developed in earth's primordial seas, they had to invent means of keeping themselves separate from the rest of the soup of organic material around them. From this need, presumably, the immunologic system arose.

The first organisms were made from the materials in that soup, yet had to segregate themselves from it. Failure to do so would have been as disastrous as an automobile assembly line in which each new car attracted to itself, indiscriminately, all the steel, glass and rubber in its vicinity.

Even today we all face that same problem. The things we eat, drink, and touch, the germs that live in us, on us, and around us—all have chemical characteristics much like the tissues of our own bodies. We must have ways of telling the foreign from the native.

"The immunologic process is our license to live in the sea of micro-organisms and as individuals anywhere," says Dr. Robert A. Good, president of Sloan-Kettering Institute for Cancer Research in New York.

It is also becoming clear that derangements of the system are a major cause of illness. It is estimated that at any one time there are between 10 million and 20 million Americans who have diseases in which immunologic mechanisms play a major role. The figure becomes much higher than that if everyone with an allergy is included, because allergies are classic cases of the immunologic system gone awry.

There are many diseases in which immunology is probably a factor because the system acts too little, too late, too much or in the wrong way. There is an impressive list of illnesses in which this is suspected: some of heart and kidney disease, much of arthritis and related conditions, and perhaps all of cancer.

There are also scores of rare diseases with such names as *Wiskott-Aldrich syndrome, Swiss-type agammaglobulinemia* and *systemic lupus erythematosis* that reflect either deficiencies or derangements of the system.

The fact that so much of human illness has some immunologic component is one reason for the current interest, but more important, from a practical viewpoint, is the incredible precision of the immunologic language and the rapidly accumulating understanding of how it works. These, together, offer the hope of influencing the system in precise ways to achieve a desired effect without doing damage to anything else.

For example, it should be possible to use the system to attack cancer cells in a patient's body while having no effect at all on closely related normal cells of the same organ in the same person. This is still beyond practical possibility, but well within the bounds of theory. Current treatment methods are much blunter, killing some normal cells as well as those of the cancer. Success, at present, depends on a hazardous balance between damage to the patient and damage to the cancer.

Another area of high current excitement centers on experiments showing that hereditary immunologic traits are probably an important factor in determining how susceptible any person may be to a given type of disease.

The evidence for this has been accumulating rapidly.

Much of it was summarized in a recent article in *Science* by Drs. Baruj Benacerraf of the Harvard Medical School and Dr. Hugh O. McDevitt, of Stanford University's School of Medicine.

In mice and guinea pigs, and probably in other species including man, the genetics of the susceptibility to disease are linked closely to those genes that put an individual signature on every person's tissues. Those are the signatures that create the main problems for the surgeon who wants to transplant a kidney or a heart from one person to another.

During a recent interview, Dr. McDevitt said that this kind of information could be used to help sort people out according to the diseases most likely to afflict them in the future—provided considerable amounts of money were made available to do the necessary surveys and other studies.

Even without this kind of major effort, he said, the new understanding of the links between the genetics of the immune system and the genetics of disease susceptibility could tell scientists much about the way diseases arise in man.

The research also merges into another of the key issues of current immunology: the functions of the main cells of the immunologic system and the dialogue among them.

In particular this involves two general populations of lymphoid cells called T cells (for thymus, a little gland high in the chest) and B cells (for bone marrow).

Their existence and roles as separate populations in the body have only come to light within the last few years, and they are the subject of much current debate.

There are many ways in which greater knowledge of T cell and B cell functions and their interactions could be applied for the benefit of human health. There appear to be conditions in which it would be helpful to turn up the dial, so to speak, on one or the other cell population while leaving the other alone. There are also unwanted immunologic responses that might be blocked without damaging the rest of the body's internal defense system by manipulation of either T or B cells—if one knew how to do it.

One of the most obvious cases is that of transplantation, whether it be a heart, kidney, liver or a piece of skin. In all of these operations the main problem is not surgical technique but coming to terms with the body's jealous guard over its own individuality.

The immune system desperately resists the presence of any foreign tissue. To keep the transplanted organ from being destroyed, surgeons must give their patients powerful drugs that suppress much of the immunological system— and thus often put the transplant recipient at risk of infectious disease.

If T cells alone could be suppressed, the problem would be much simplified because they seem to be the main agents of tissue immunity.

It appears that the precursors of both cell populations form in the bone marrow—the source of blood and much of the body's immunologic capabilities. The T cells then pass through and are influenced by the thymus, which proves to be one of the body's main immunological organs.

While T cells are so-called because of their link to the thymus, B cells get their name not only from the bone marrow derivation but also from the fact that they seem comparable to immunologically active cells in fowl that come from an organ near the tail called the *Bursa of Fabricius*. Experts are still searching today for the equivalent of the bursa in man.

Dr. Good, whose research at the University of Minnesota developed much of current knowledge of the thymus and its role, thinks that the human bursa equivalent possibly may only appear briefly in the individual's development and then regress, leaving no trace sufficient for its identification.

At present it appears that the T cells are the main agents of cellular immunity—the kind that resists tissue transplantation and is responsible for important kinds of allergic reactions.

T cells are capable of destructive action when they encounter something they don't like. They also seem capable of mobilizing the scavenger cells called "macrophages" at the scene of action so that they can swallow enemies detected by the other immunologic cells.

It is widely suspected that T cell antipathy to the foreign is an important bulwark against the cancer cells in the body and that this probably has its roots deep in evolution as a defense of "self" against anything extraneous.

As scientists interpret the picture now, humoral immunity—the system that involves circulating antibodies—is a key factor in preventing infection. Once an infection is actually started, perhaps because the antibody system was

41

not yet primed to prevent it, a key force in recovery is the cellular immunity system based largely on the cooperative action of T cells and B cells.

But this is a two-edged sword. Sometimes the T cells are tricked into enmity toward normal constituents of the individual's body. Self-destructive immune effects then produce something called autoimmune disease. Scientists think it probable that this is the key problem in many important maladies such as rheumatoid arthritis, rheumatic heart disease and some destructive kinds of kidney disease, as well as in other less familiar types of serious illness.

B cells on the other hand, are the precursors of the cells that make antibodies, the globular proteins found in the blood that seem to be a main defense against germs.

There is some evidence that certain viruses—including those that cause flu and some animal cancers—are resisted mainly by B cell functions, while fungus diseases and some bacteria, including those of typhoid and tuberculosis, lie more in the province of the T cell.

But the picture emerging today in laboratories throughout the world is far more complicated and significant than that. Much of the current excitement and debate is on the way the populations of cells communicate with one another and trigger into activity any of several kinds of immune response.

Antibodies, themselves produced on the orders of B cells, invoke the aid of a whole family of substances named "complement" which generate a whole cascade of reactions to deal with anything the antibody points out as dangerous.

Some experts believe there may well be several types of T cells, each with its own special functions.

The whole immunologic system appears to use all of these cells and proteins in an arrangement of checks and balances, signals, countersignals, and duplicate defenses that must have arisen and proliferated through evolution because life depended on them.

While T and B cells each have separate functions, it is becoming clear that they work most effectively together. Study of this cooperation is one of the hottest areas of current immunological research. Any gathering of immunologists is likely to erupt into a debate over the nature and significance of the signals that pass between T cells and B cells.

It is clear that the system must tell the body to tolerate some things and reject many others. Too jealous a guard by the defense system can lead to over-reaction and even self-destruction—precisely what seems to happen in allergic conditions and autoimmune disease.

Too lax a defense, on the other hand, can lead to infection or possibly cancer. Some scientists guess that as many as 100 or even 1,000 cancer cells arise by accident in any normal person every day but are destroyed.

Dr. Melvin Cohn, a senior fellow of the Salk Institute for Biological Studies at La Jolla, Calif., describes the immunologic system as walking a tightrope continuously to tolerate the harmless and yet react destructively against the potentially dangerous.

In this he sees the cooperation of T and B cells as vital. In his view the system works a little like the safeguards that the government has developed to prevent any mistaken triggering of a nuclear weapons assault. It takes more than one signal from more than one individual to fire the missiles.

According to Dr. Cohn's theory, one signal from an immunologically active cell spells tolerance. Two simultaneous signals start the war.

Dr. Richard Dutton of The University of California at San Diego has been searching for some chemical messenger, released by T cells, that carries the signal to the B cell. He and others consider the triggering mechanism, whatever it proves to be, as one of the most exciting areas of search.

Dr. Uhr, now at Baylor University, has described the triggering event as akin to the ringing of a doorbell.

Whatever it is, the signaling is a reaction to the body's encounter with something called an "antigen." This is really just a name for anything that the body is capable of recognizing as foreign. The signaling that achieves this recognition is probably more easily described in terms of braille than spoken language. The recognition is a matter of shape. The business end of the antigen fits, in lock-and-key fashion, a receptor on the surface of the cell.

When this process sounds the alarm, the scavenger cells called macrophages may be drawn to the site. T cells with destructive capabilities may multiply and attack, and B cells may be stimulated to make antibody.

This latter part of the process is as remarkable as any.

Scientists generally believe today that the individual

is endowed from the start with a whole library of receptors on his B cells, one or more of which is capable of fitting the shape of any antigen that may be encountered during life.

It is a little like giving a tourist a key to the city, except that it is not just one key nor was it cut deliberately to fit any one lock. Instead, it is as though some key-maker ground out keys in every shape he could imagine, confident that somewhere there would be a lock to fit it. This appears to be the way the immunologic system prepares to make antibodies that will fit any antigen the body will ever encounter.

Once triggered, an antibody-producing cell makes antibodies in profusion, each cell producing only one specific type. Since some scientists estimate there are as many as a trillion precursors of antibody-producing cells in a normal human being, this gives a broad enough range of shapes to meet the need.

In recent years, much has been learned about the antibodies themselves. They are molecules of a type of protein called immunoglobulin, and at least five major types are known.

Among these are immunoglobulin G—the circulating antibody active against bacteria, viruses, and foreign proteins; immunoglobulin A, secreted in the nose, respiratory and digestive tracts and at other places to give local protection against invasion; immunoglobulin M, which appears to be the first antibody formed to deal with any newly recognized antigen, and immunoglobulin E, which has recently been identified as the type that figures in allergic reactions. Although the fifth type, immunoglobulin D, has been detected, its functions are still unknown.

A recent finding that may prove to be of critical importance was the discovery that people who respond poorly to an antigen, mobilize their antibodies against it in an abnormal way. They seem unable to switch properly from making IgM to making IgG. Why this is so is not yet understood, but it could help explain the puzzle of some individuals' poor resistance to certain infections. For the long-term it suggests a strategy for coping with that lack of resistance. Such items as this show why there is so much current interest in the study of antibodies, but even though much has been learned in recent years it is only a beginning.

Antibodies have been harvested, tagged, analyzed, and even photographed. Dr. Gerald M. Edelman and colleagues at Rockefeller University have actually deciphered the complete chemical structure of an immunoglobulin G molecule, the most prevalent of the antibody types known in man. Dr. Edelman was awarded a Nobel Prize in 1972 for his research on antibodies.

The basic antibody structure is known to consist of four chains of chemical subunits—two light chains and two heavy chains. On these are large "constant regions" that are the same from antibody to antibody and appear to dictate function. There are also variable regions that confer specificity— the combining sites of the antibodies. The variability itself —the factor that allows antibodies to be formed to fit any conceivable antigen—seems to result from genetic mutation in the producing cell. There is still no complete explanation of that variability, however, and no consensus among scientists on how it is arranged.

Armed with so much knowledge of the nature of antibodies and the cells that produce them, some scientists, such as Dr. John Fahey of the University of California at Los Angeles, are trying to grow them artificially in the laboratory. He and his colleagues have human cells growing in laboratory flasks that do make immunoglobulin but, so far as they can tell, it is not actually antibody to any known antigen.

If specific human antibodies could be made, the potential for their use, both in research and for medical purposes, would be vast, Dr. Fahey noted during an interview.

No one thinks that goal is just around the corner, but there is no reason to think it is forever out of reach either. Chemists have already demonstrated that it is possible to synthesize enzymes from the appropriate amino acid building blocks. If this can be done for enzymes, why not, eventually, for antibodies?

Taken together, all of several lines of research related to antibodies hint at the possibility of a whole new era of passive immunization. In its obvious and familiar form, passive immunization means giving the patient gamma globulin to protect temporarily against an infectious disease. The antibodies, also known as immunoglobulins, are found in the gamma globulin fraction of blood. Thus, passive immunization is really the act of borrowing antibodies from one person to give short term protection to another.

The method is sometimes used to prevent—or at least to ameliorate—a hepatitis infection in a person who has just been exposed to the disease. In the days before the development of polio vaccines, gamma globulin was used quite widely to protect close relatives of polio victims.

But the limitations of the method are obvious. Gamma globulin is a relatively scarce commodity, since the only source is human blood. It isn't universally effective and, in some cases, can interfere with the development of lasting immunity.

If laboratory-grown—or tailor-made—antibodies could ever be produced, the possibilities of passive immunization would be broadened greatly. Antibodies that are rare at present might become available in wholesale lots. Perhaps antibodies more potent and specific than the natural varieties might be made. There might also be other research and treatment uses yet to be imagined. Predictions of this sort are hazardous in a field as complex and as fast moving as immunology.

Altogether, the complexity of the immunologic system seems to rival that of any other body system with the possible exception of the brain. And some scientists see links between the brain and the immunologic system as being potentially highly rewarding to study.

In the case of immunology, the complexity of the system is an irresistible challenge to scientific curiosity. But it is also more than that.

The very fact of such complexity means that there ought to be many points within the system at which a person who knows enough could apply leverage to make a change. Many who specialize in immunology believe it offers medicine and science an almost infinite array of opportunities against many of mankind's worst afflictions.

3

THE ANARCHIST
WITHIN

IN mice and guinea pigs, scientists have been able to
make cancers diminish or even fade away by deliberately
manipulating the animals' own natural immunologic defenses.

Why can't they do the same thing in humans?

It is a question that any of the 650,000 Americans who
will discover they have cancer this year might justifiably
ask.

There is no simple or single answer, but there is a vast
search under way. Doctors in the United States and abroad
are already testing new immunologic methods of cancer
treatment in small numbers of patients, slowly working
through several strategies suggested by basic research.

Some are trying to increase the vigor of the patient's
immunologic defenses in general. Others are specifically
trying to make cancer tissue more "visible" and provocative
to the patient's defense system. Still others are trying to
borrow immunologically active cells or other materials
from a person thought to have defenses already alerted
against the patient's kind of cancer.

Many of these attempts are just beginning. Some have
histories that go back several years. Most have yet to prove

their value. But interest among specialists has been growing. If there is a way to overcome cancer, many believe, at least part of it will be found in immunology.

The immunological system is natural, powerful, and wonderfully discriminative. It can differentiate among the three types of polio virus or the many types and subtypes of human blood. Impressive data have been amassed indicating it can discriminate between cancer cells and normal cells living side by side in a patient's tissues.

Capable of such fine distinctions, the system would seem a logical way of giving doctors the means to kill cancer cells within a patient while leaving normal cells unharmed. In theory it should be a powerful tool for early diagnosis and even prevention. These possibilities are the promise of the field, and evidence is growing to support them. But today that promise is still largely unfulfilled.

The body's natural immunological defenses have, for years, tantalized doctors by their glimmer of hope for cancer treatment. The first such attempts were made before the turn of the present century. Apparently they all failed. No one really knew enough about the forces they were trying to manipulate. Probably they still don't know enough, but specialists in all the fields that bear on immunology are learning fast.

The system would seem to be a natural choice for a weapon against cancer. There have been a few thoroughly documented cases in man in which malignant tumors have simply faded away and vanished. Sometimes these disappearances have followed infection or other events that might jolt the immune defense system into heightened activity. The most plausible explanation is that somehow, the balance between tumor and defenses shifted and the defenses won. So far as is known, this happens only rarely with established tumors and why that should be true is a mystery in itself.

Research during the past decade has established firmly the principle that cancers in animals are antigenic to their hosts. That is, the cancerous cell will have new antigens on its surface that the animal's immune defenses can recognize as foreign. There is little if any doubt that the same thing is true in man. The human cancer cell will have specific antigens not present on normal cells of the same kind of tissue.

So the early attempts at cancer immunotherapy can be justified logically, but the results were dismal. Cancer vaccines of various types were tried and failed. Most other attempts to bolster the patient's natural defenses were wholly disappointing. Some prominent specialists have viewed the whole field with frank disfavor.

"Immunology was almost a dirty word in cancer," one scientist and administrator said recently.

But, today, the situation is far different. Dr. Frank J. Rauscher, Jr., director of the newly-expanded National Cancer Institute, has said repeatedly that he considers immunology one of the brightest long-range hopes of the cancer research field. The men and women who are doing that research know far more about the body's natural defenses than they did just a few years ago. The main classes of immunologically active cells and their functions are far better understood than heretofore.

The lymphocytes—T cells and B cells—can be taken together as one of those classes although each of these co-operating cell types has distinctive functions of its own.

The T cells are sometimes involved in direct attack on anything they perceive as "the enemy." Probably, part of their natural role is that of surveillance against cancer cells arising in the body spontaneously from time to time.

If the T cells could be persuaded to react more powerfully against cancer cells that have already gained a foothold, they might contribute to cure as well as prevention. In fact, there is recent evidence that some strategies already employed to combat cancer with immunology may, unwittingly, be doing so through the T cells. One of the current strategies is to use substances called adjuvants to heighten the effectiveness of anticancer treatment. Fundamentally, these are substances which, when injected with an antigen, will increase the immune response to that antigen. There are many kinds of adjuvants, some of which have been used medically for many years. Among them are water in oil emulsions, alum precipitates, and the anti-tuberculosis vaccine BCG (for Bacillus Calmette-Guerin) of which we will hear more later.

The new data indicates that many adjuvants enhance immunity specifically by increasing the activity of T cells. Some experts say there is a prime need at present to learn more about how adjuvants work and to develop better ones.

Evidently, the B cells are affected little if at all by adjuvants. Nevertheless, these cells—precursors of anti-body-forming cells—might also be mobilized more effectively against cancer if anyone could figure out just how to do it. Attempts to produce antibodies were among the earliest efforts to attack cancer through immunology. But present understanding of the problem shows serious hazards in this approach. Antibodies can indirectly enhance a cancer's growth as well as help destroy it.

The other main class of cells in the immunologic arsenal is made up of histiocytes and macrophages. Each type, in its own way, can be a killer. The histiocytes seem to work their destructive effects by some action against the surface of the cells they attack. The macrophages literally engulf the enemy.

Scientists at Oak Ridge National Laboratory have recently taken pictures under the microscope showing these killer cells in action against cancer cells. Under their assault, the cancer cells seem to be deteriorating.

But in animals with experimental cancers and in cancer patients there is much evidence that the immune defenses are not functioning normally. Patients whose cancers are growing progressively tend to have somewhat lower than normal numbers of lymphocytes. Such patients seem to have reduced ability to be sensitized by, and to react against, chemicals that ordinarily provoke reactions. Skin tests involving common bacteria also give poor reactions in these people.

Animal research suggests that these are all effects of the very presence of a mass of tumor tissue, and that they don't necessarily imply a basic fault in the immune defenses. This is hopeful because it suggests that just the right nudge to the system, coupled with just the right attack on the cancer, might shift the balance back from defeat to victory.

At the same time, it has been widely observed that persons who have basic immunologic deficiencies and those who must take drugs that suppress their immune systems have a greater than average risk of cancer. These facts stand as complementary evidence that immunology is a key to the problem.

The question is how to grasp that key and the question is a huge one. While it is far from answered, there is emerging a general picture of the way the great defense system functions in the normal person and under the assault of cancer.

From this picture, in turn, new ideas are emerging for intervention against malignant disease.

The body of fact and theory that has refocused so much attention on the immunology of cancer was summarized recently by Dr. Richard T. Smith of the University of Florida, Gainesville. In his view, the basic points that have emerged after years of study in men and animals are these:

Generally, animal and human cancer cells have new surface antigens that are recognizably foreign to the body in which they grow.

In normal individuals, the immunologic defense system carries on continual surveillance to detect such danger signs of foreignness and to destroy any cells on which such signs arise.

Once cancer cells escape surveillance and become established as a tumor, parts of the immunologic system become weak or completely ineffective.

After it has started to grow, a cancer deluges the body with a continuous rain of tumor cells and fragments. Many specialists believe this shower of cells and debris overwhelms the defense system.

Every part of the defense system that reacts against foreign tissues also reacts against these cancer cells; but, paradoxically, the tumor and the defenses can coexist without destruction of the cancer.

This is the essential picture, parts of it still subject to considerable debate, that is coming into focus in what appears to be a new era in immunologic research on cancer.

This branch of biological science has already become an almost universal tool for seeking knowledge of the nature of cancer cells and their relations with the rest of the body. Immunologic tests are crucial to the widespread search for viruses that may be among the causes of human cancer.

Early diagnosis seems a logical target for a system that appears capable of distinguishing cancer cells from normal ones. If different cancers shed clues to their existence in the blood stream, this too should be valuable.

At present the candidate some scientists consider most promising for an early diagnostic test is something called

CEA—for carcino-embryonic antigen. It was discovered in the mid-nineteen sixties by Dr. Phil Gold and co-workers at McGill University, Montreal. Now under study at many centers, it was first thought to occur only in normal embryonic tissue and in cancers of the colon.

It has since been detected in other cancer tissues too. At present its main potential seems to be that of gauging the response to treatment of a person known to have cancer, but some experts still hope for a larger role.

Beyond the uses of immunology in basic research and in diagnosis, there is new enthusiasm for its possibilities in the treatment of patients for whom conventional means have failed.

There appear to be at least twenty medical teams here and abroad making such attempts, according to Dr. William D. Terry, chief of the National Cancer Institute's immunology branch. Fundamentally, the doctors are trying a sort of biochemical judo—using characteristics of the cancer against itself and trying, by related means, to strengthen the patient's resistance to his or her own disease. There are several basic strategies. In a recent publication, Drs. Herbert F. Oettgen, Lloyd J. Old and Edward A. Boyse of Sloan-Kettering Institute in New York summarized some that have been tried or considered.

These include attempts to immunize the patient with cancer cells or extracts; to borrow someone else's immunity by transfusion of lymphocytes, their extracts, or other materials; to transfer specific cell-killing antibodies from one person to another; to treat the patient with agents that stimulate general immunologic reactivity such as the chemical called DNCB or the tuberculosis vaccine BCG.

"There are pitfalls in each of these conventional approaches," the authors noted, "and none has yet been shown unequivocally to alter the course of human cancer in a predictable fashion."

Some new variations on the theme of using general immunological stimulators such as BCG are just beginning. Although they can show no definitive results yet, some have already made a dramatic difference for a few patients.

For example, at a scientific meeting in 1972, a doctor showed a series of photographs of a breast cancer patient whose disease had reappeared as an ugly cancerous sore at the site of an amputated breast. Pictures taken during and after the treatment with BCG showed the cancer dwindling progressively and the sore healing.

The specialist who showed the photographs, Dr. Edmund Klein of Roswell Park Memorial Institute in Buffalo, emphasized that he was not claiming this recurrent cancer was cured. He does claim to have given the patient a lengthy respite from pain and discomfort.

Through this case and several others in a series of more than two dozen, he also claims to have demonstrated the possibilities of a strategy for cancer treatment widely believed to have great potential—in those patients who can be induced to respond.

This is the strategy of producing, in the vicinity of the cancer, the cellular immunologic reaction called delayed hypersensitivity. This is of the same basic type as the poison ivy reaction although more drastic.

To do this, Dr. Klein applies to the cancer site something known to produce this kind of reaction. One such substance is the compound DNCB. Another, which figures importantly in cancer research today, is BCG.

The belief is that the stimulation provokes a heightened allergic reaction and that this helps the body react powerfully against the cancer tissue as well.

During a period of several years, Dr. Klein has demonstrated that his approach is highly effective against skin cancer and may have some preventive action against its recurrence as well. Several other medical centers have adopted the method.

But skin cancer remains a special case. Will the method work against cancers that are remote and inaccessible? The results in some breast cancer cases and others suggest that it will, but the cases have been few and only some of those have responded favorably.

In research with guinea pigs, Dr. Herbert J. Rapp of the National Cancer Institute, and colleagues have provided strong evidence that Dr. Klein's basic strategy is valid. Some experts believe that the research at the Cancer Institute has provided the first clear-cut animal model of immunotherapy, something highly important to future progress in the field.

Dr. Georges Mathé of the Hôpital Paul-Brousse near Paris is using BCG to prolong the outwardly disease-free "remission" period in some patients with acute leukemia.

Dr. Mathé uses conventional drug treatment to reduce the number of cancer cells to as small a number as possible and then treats the patient with BCG scratched into the skin. At the same time the patient receives chemically killed cancer cells injected at a site different from that of the BCG.

In some patients, this treatment has significantly prolonged the period of remission from the disease. Some of these remissions have already lasted several months and are still in effect.

But the research has also demonstrated that only some acute leukemia patients will respond. For others it does not seem to help. Furthermore, the method depends on conventional drug treatment to produce remission in the first place.

Dr. Donald L. Morton of the University of California at Los Angeles and Dr. Hilliard F. Seigler of Duke University have, independently of each other, produced strikingly long remissions of several years from malignant melanoma, a cancer of black pigment-forming cells, by treatment methods that involve direct injection of BCG into the tumor site.

The total number of patients followed long enough for evaluation in both series is still small. In terms of more widespread cancer treatment, the significance is obviously hopeful but still unclear. One difficulty is that melanoma is highly variable and capricious. It can flare up or subside unpredictably for no obvious reason.

It seems firmly established that BCG can stimulate the body's immunological defense system against a cancer—if there is still enough of the system functioning to respond to it. But the evidence to date suggests that this is by no means always the case.

There are also other methods of making a cancer more "visible" and provocative to the immunologic system. One, of particular current interest, is to treat cancer cells with an enzyme, called a neuraminidase, produced by the bacteria that cause cholera.

Two groups of scientists have each demonstrated that mice can be cured of solid cancers when the enzyme is used to increase the "immunogenicity"—or immunologic "visibility"—of the cancer tissue.

Reports on this have been published recently by Dr. Richard L. Simmons of the University of Minnesota School of Medicine; and Drs. J. George Bekesi and James F. Holland and their colleagues at Roswell Park Memorial Institute.

The strategy is to treat cancer cells with the enzyme to heighten their "visibility," treat them also with another substance to insure that they will not grow—and then inject them into the animal in which the same type of cancer is growing.

Dr. Simmons has observed that about a third of the animals treated in this way then react against their cancers and destroy them. The effect appears to be specific for the types of cancer cell used to stimulate the immune defenses. A different type of cancer growing in the same animal will not by destroyed.

Recently Dr. Simmons has begun trying the method in a

few carefully selected patients. In answer to a question, he said that the treatment looks promising but that it is far too early to tell how useful it will be.

Another new strategy for cancer treatment stems from research done in recent years by scientists at the University of Washington School of Medicine in Seattle.

The key figures in this work are a husband and wife team. Dr. Karl E. and Ingegerd Hellstrom and a colleague, Dr. Hans Olov Sjogren.

In a field already plagued by paradoxes, they found one that many scientists consider particularly important. The immunologic defense system, in man and animals, appeared to be producing a specific something that actually prevented other elements of the system from attacking a growing cancer.

This was most clearly demonstrated by research in the test tube. Individuals in whom cancer was growing had in their circulations immunologically active lymphocytes that would destroy the cancer cells in laboratory tests, but not in their bodies. The reason became clear when serum from such a person was put in the same test tube with the lymphocytes and the cancer cells. Something in the serum blocked the destructive action of the lymphocytes.

The Hellstroms have called this "blocking antibody" or, alternatively, "blocking factor."

In patients, the scientists in Seattle have discovered that the blocking antibody—or factor—appears in the blood serum before the cancer takes a demonstrable turn for the worse; and that it is undetectable in cancers that have been brought under control by surgery, radiation or other means.

This suggests that periodic tests for blocking factor in a patient's serum might be valuable in gauging how well he or she was responding to cancer treatment. An obvious further suggestion is that some kind of action to remove or inactivate blocking factor might be a valuable treatment in itself.

A more recent although controversial finding by the group in Seattle has an even more direct application. Their new evidence indicates that the cancer patient's body can also produce an antidote to the blocking factor—something they now call "un-blocking antibody."

They have produced some evidence that this can help an animal fight its cancer and, recently, they have begun the cautious application of this approach to a few selected patients.

The "un-blocking" serum would come from patients whose cancers appeared to have been cured or arrested. The cancers would have to be of the same type as those of the patients to be treated. The plan is to try the method in five patients the first year and then expand the effort if it seems warranted.

As yet, of course, no one knows whether this strategy will be useful. The Hellstroms emphasize that they do not consider it ready yet for any use in patients except in the course of a careful study and evaluation on a research basis. There are potential dangers as well as potential benefits in any new treatment.

All of the new methods of immunotherapy represent

ventures to the edge of the unknown. They rest on the mass of basic scientific information that has been gathered in recent years and presumably will contribute to it as well.

But while the applications must rest on the scientific base, the attempts to apply this knowledge involve difficult technical, and sometimes ethical and legal problems.

Progress can only be made by confronting these problems.

"All of these methods are likely to fail, but they have to be tried," said one cancer specialist with a blend of pessimism and implied hope that is typical of his field.

What he meant was basically this: Cancer is not only a grave health problem, but one of the most difficult and complicated mysteries of biology. It is entwined everywhere with the fundamentals of life itself.

Only by exploring those new leads that appear promising can theories be tested and pieces of the mystery be chipped away. Thus, the defeats of today and tomorrow may reveal the path to a victory thereafter; and no one has any way of knowing how far—or how close—"thereafter" may prove to be.

4

GIFTS OF LIFE

T

HEY are as various as humanity itself, but they all have something desperately important in common. They are all living on time borrowed with living tissues from someone else.

These are the several thousand men, women, and children whose lives have been saved, at least for the time being, by transplantation. They are all beneficiaries of that same rapidly advancing realm of science that is crucial to many aspects of human health—immunology.

It is in fact the immune system that finally determines the success or failure of a transplant. Whether the new organ is a heart, liver, or kidney, the body's normal internal defenses respond by attacking and destroying it because the body sees the transplant as foreign. The assault is implacable and deadly.

Indeed there have been many failures. Transplants are successful only because doctors have found ways to call a truce with the immunological defenses. But the truce is imperfect and often just temporary. Research teams in laboratories throughout the world are trying to improve that situation—to make the truce more dependable and even to achieve a lasting peace between the transplanted organ and its new owner.

But, today each success still represents a life that almost wasn't saved—and is still hostage to possible destruction by the body's immunological defenses.

Among the case histories is a housewife from England who was dying of incurable liver disease more than three years ago and now, to all outward appearances, is in good health. She owes this to the gift of a liver from a young boy who was killed in an auto accident.

Another is an interior decorator in California whose every pulse for the past three and a half years has come from the beating of a heart that used to belong to someone else—again an accident victim.

More typical are the several thousand kidney transplant patients—a physician from the Punjab, a teenage girl from Connecticut, a telephone operator in Arlington, Va. who also finds time to be a television repairman and member of a bowling team. In 1963 doctors told him his death was "just a matter of time."

Far from typical, but important scientifically, is the case of a young man from a farm in Indiana. In the spring of 1971 he was dying of aplastic anemia, an illness in which the patient's bone marrow stops functioning, thus virtually halting his production of blood. The usual end-result is death from hemorrhage or infection.

Conventional treatment with drugs had failed, and the patient was near death when doctors at the University of Washington in Seattle gave him a transplant of bone marrow from his sister. Nearly two years later the doctors were still able to report that their patient was alive, evidently healthy, and with no sign of his "fatal" anemia. But the blood that flows in his veins bears all the traits of his sister's blood and none of his own.

Transplant patients and their immunological problems have been of particular interest recently for reasons of both science and economics. Changes in the Social Security law, that became effective on July 1, 1973, gave Medicare coverage to workers of any age, or their dependents, who require kidney transplants or regular treatment by artificial kidney machine. Both immediately and in the long run, this is expected to increase the number of transplants that are performed. The number is already large.

An international registry maintained jointly by the American College of Surgeons and the National Institutes of Health showed that more than 11,000 kidneys had been transplanted altogether by the end of 1972. Of these, 4,500 —nearly half of the total number ever transplanted—were functioning at that time and keeping their recipients alive. New kidney transplants are being done now at a rate of almost 3,000 a year. The figure for 1972 was 2,900.

Considering that the overall survival figures include the early days of transplantation, when the normal expectation was failure, current totals are impressive.

The transplant numbers for other organs are far smaller, but include some dramatic successes such as the four heart transplant patients who have each survived into the fifth year of borrowed life and the five liver transplant patients who passed the one-year mark.

All of these represent partial triumphs over the immunological defense system and evidence that lives can be saved long before the last scientific word is written on the subject.

The purely surgical problems of transplantation were solved long ago. The remaining great barrier is immunological.

Although immunosuppressive drugs have made modern transplantation possible, some experts believe that these chemicals cannot carry progress much further. Scientists are searching for ways of making the body tolerate a transplant without drugs and for better ways of matching the recipient with the best potential donor.

Specific tolerance, the holy grail of the transplantation immunologist, is a state in which the person who has received a new organ such as a heart or a kidney would simply accept it as "self" and not be forever imperiled by the threat of rejection.

This has been achieved experimentally in animals, but not—at least not intentionally—in man. Indeed, the very concept of immunological tolerance has come under debate in recent months.

"There is occurring a radical restructuring of our understanding of immunological tolerance," said a recent report from the National Institute of Allergy and Infectious Diseases.

The classic view is that the "tolerant" individual simply does not have the capacity to recognize the specific transplanted tissue as foreign. More recent evidence suggests that the tolerant body still has immunologically active cells that could attack the foreign tissue but that they are prevented from doing so by an active blocking mechanism.

This issue is still unsettled. Evidence supporting each concept was presented at the Fourth International Congress of the Transplantation Society.

Experts at that meeting said it was likely that both concepts were right in a sense—that unresponsiveness in the classic sense could exist under some circumstances and that blocking of the immunological attack might protect a transplant in others.

Dr. Paul Russell of Harvard Medical School, president of the Transplantation Society in 1972, saw evidence in patients he and his colleagues have studied that suggests tolerance is a rational goal. Repeated tests of long-term kidney transplant survivors show that some of them become less and less reactive to their transplants with the passage of time, he said.

What relation these cases bear to true tolerance in the classic sense is unclear, but they offer hope through the implication that something that occurs naturally might, in the future, be achieved by design.

A recent report by scientists at the University of California at Los Angeles runs counter to classic theory in a related matter involving the response of the body to repeated transplants.

The scientists, Drs. Gerhard Opelz, Max R. Mickey, and Paul I. Terasaki studied the data from several hundred cases in the United States and abroad in which patients received second kidney transplants after first ones had been rejected. Classical theory, they noted, would have predicted rejection of the second kidney at least as rapidly and probably more rapidly than the first.

In fact, however, there was one group of patients whose second transplants survived significantly longer than the first. They were individuals whose first transplants were rejected slowly over the course of several months.

The doctors concluded that these patients' immunologic reactions to the first transplant were somehow conditioning their bodies to be more receptive to the second.

One obvious implication is that if this was indeed happening and if the mechanism could be thoroughly understood it might be possible to do it on purpose for the patients' benefit. Even if that did not prove practical, the ability to predict which patients would or would not react in this way would be valuable.

One major thrust in transplantation research during the last decade has been the effort to define human solid tissue types in a way analogous to blood types. Other means of matching the tissues of donors and recipients have also been sought to minimize the rejection problem.

The ideal case is a transplant from one of a pair of identical twins to the other. Their tissues are genetically the same. There is no immunologic barrier between them.

In fact, kidney transplants from twin to twin, starting in

1954, gave the field the initial successes on which everything since has rested.

But transplantation would have remained a curiosity of no real medical importance if it had not been possible to expand its usefulness beyond identical twins. Hence the interest in immunosuppressive drugs and ways of typing and matching tissues.

The typing system most widely used today has been developed over a period of almost a decade through the contributions of many scientists here and abroad. It is called the HL-A system, a designation some scientists say derives from the words *Human Leukocyte Antigen*. Leukocytes are white blood cells, and they are thought to have all the markers of tissue types that are found in solid tissues.

HL-A typing is done by a series of blood tests, but the system has proved to be far more complex than the universally used ABO system of red blood cell types. After all the time and international effort devoted to the system, it still appears to have some serious limitations. There is considerable debate over its usefulness in predicting the success of a transplant between two unrelated persons.

Dr. Jean Dausset, of the University of Paris, a major figure in European tissue typing and a principal pioneer in developing the system, says it is of value. His substantial data from European transplant work show that the better the match in tissue type, the better the chance of success.

But equally impressive data from Dr. Terasaki's laboratory at U.C.L.A., where most tissue typing in the United

States is done, tells a different story. He says there is a strong correlation when donor and recipient are close relatives. A perfect, or nearly perfect match, almost always predicts success.

But, among unrelated persons he finds little or no correlation. A good match in tissue types does not necessarily predict a good result, nor a bad match a poor one.

There is no obvious explanation for the fact that Dr. Dausset's reports of kidney transplants in Europe give the HL-A system higher marks than Dr. Terasaki's data in the United States. But even those who believe the system will ultimately prove sufficient, concede that it is not so at present. Some believe the HL-A system of tissue typing will prove to be only the tip of the immunologic iceberg.

Dr. Fritz H. Bach, his wife Marilyn, and their colleagues at the University of Wisconsin think HL-A typing misses some important things for reasons to be found in recently discovered details concerning the immunological defense system. Their studies in carefully inbred strains of mice suggest that the two main classes of immunologically active cells—the T cells and the B cells "see" things in somewhat different ways.

The B cells, being the precursors of antibody-forming cells, would detect the tissue type markers that are detectable through the blood tests used in the HL-A system. This is reasonable because, in general, the antibodies circulate in the blood.

But the T cells, too, are key factors in the immunological defenses and can set in motion a chain of events capable of destroying transplanted tissue. If the T cells "view" of things is not represented in the current blood tests, this would leave important gaps in the tissue profile that the typing tests reveal.

These gaps are presumably not so important in matching two closely related persons. Tissue types are determined by heredity. It seems reasonable to expect that, in the case of a brother and sister who are perfect HL-A matches, the unknown factors also match because they are carried along in the process of heredity. When unrelated persons are involved, there is no reason why this should happen.

Evidence that there is indeed a difference between the significance of perfect matches in siblings—brother or sister—and in the nonrelated pairs comes from a field of transplantation that is considered particularly important today. This is bone marrow transplantation—in a sense, the ultimate transplant, because bone marrow is the key immunologic tissue.

A group led by Dr. E. Donnall Thomas at the University of Washington, Seattle, has achieved some remarkable successes recently with bone marrow transplants in which the donor-recipient pairs were siblings who matched perfectly in terms of both the HL-A system and another widely used test called the mixed leukocyte culture test.

But there were failures even among these seemingly perfectly matched pairs. Furthermore, Dr. Thomas has said that he knows of no case in which a bone marrow transplant was successful when the match was less than perfect.

In most persons other than identical twins a bone marrow transplant is an all-or-nothing situation because failure of a marrow transplant means death for the patient.

As in other types of transplantation, the mechanics are relatively easy, the biology difficult and the failures at least as numerous as the successes. Marrow is taken from accessible bones in the donor's pelvis by means of a syringe. It is injected into the recipient by vein and migrates unaided to the marrow spaces of the bones where it grows and repopulates. For an adult, the amount needed for transplantation is somewhat more than a pint. This means between 10 and 20 billion marrow cells, an amount which depletes the donor of only about two percent of his total. The body probably replaces this in a day or so. The amount needed for a young child is much smaller.

In terms of delivering the material, no other type of transplant is so simple, but the problems of biology are excruciating because a marrow transplant meets the immunological barrier head on. Not only can the patient's defenses destroy the graft of marrow, but the graft can fight back and destroy its new host.

In short, the patient may die because he lacks functioning bone marrow, key tissue in blood formation, and immunological competence. He may also die because the grafted marrow, being immunologically active itself, will react against the recipient—its new host—if there is a discrepancy in tissue characteristics. This is called graft versus host disease. It is the main problem in bone marrow transplantation today.

In the Seattle group's latest reported series of eight patients given bone marrow transplants to cope with the deadly disease aplastic anemia, one died because the engrafted marrow was rejected; one died a few hours after the transplant because of a severe infection that had sent him into shock four hours before he received the new marrow; and two died of graft versus host disease, even though donor and recipient were perfectly matched according to tests available today.

Clearly, the matching is less than perfect.

The hopeful part of the story, however, concerns the four other patients treated in Seattle. At last report they were all alive and appeared to be out of danger so far as their fatal disease was concerned. Two were well into their second year. One was about to pass the first anniversary of his transplant and the fourth had passed six months. While there is no guarantee of permanent success, the crucial period is thought to be the first 100 days and all four were well beyond that.

The anemia for which they were treated involved complete failure of native marrow function, a disease that virtually halts the patient's production of blood. The usual end result is death from hemorrhage or infection.

Dr. Thomas said patients with marrow failure as complete as those almost never recover. This leaves marrow transplantation as the only hope, but he knows of no successes elsewhere to match these four.

Marrow transplantation is particularly important because in theory it could be used to treat a broad spectrum of grave illnesses and inborn defects. For medical scientists it seems likely to teach many lessons concerning immunology as well as important disease states.

The scientist from Seattle believes part of the problem for the marrow transplant patients is that most of them have received blood transfusions during the course of their treatment before a transplant was considered. He believes this may sensitize the patient and make a successful transplant more difficult.

Several of the pioneers in the field of marrow grafting, including the Seattle group and a team on the East Coast led by Dr. George Santos of Johns Hopkins University, are trying to persuade doctors to have potential bone marrow recipients typed and classified in advance to see whether a suitably matched brother or sister is available.

For those to whom this last ditch form of treatment seems both possible and warranted the strategy is to minimize blood transfusion whenever possible in the hope of giving a future marrow transplant a better chance.

Almost by definition these are all desperately sick people. There is no time to be lost. Hence the need for typing and matching in advance.

Within roughly the last two years, the Seattle group has identified twenty-six patients who might have benefited from marrow transplantation but who died before it could be done. One recent case of this sort was a boy in New

York City who was in the last stages of aplastic anemia in September 1972.

The typing and matching had been done. The donor was available. They were scheduled to fly to Seattle on a Friday. On Thursday night, only hours before they were to leave, the boy suffered a brain hemorrhage and died.

Aplastic anemia is by no means the only reason for which marrow transplantation has been attempted in man. Almost a decade ago, Dr. Georges Mathé of Hôpital Paul-Brousse obtained encouraging results in one patient using bone marrow transplantation against acute leukemia. The doctor also is reportedly doing marrow transplants for aplastic anemia with some good responses.

Leukemia is a cancer of the blood-forming tissues, of which bone marrow is the most important. It would seem a likely candidate for this kind of treatment and several medical teams have tried it.

Unfortunately there have been many cases in which the leukemia has recurred after the transplant. In two and possibly three treated by the Seattle group, the leukemia has appeared in the transplanted marrow itself weeks or months after the transplant.

Altogether, according to a report to a meeting of the International Society for Experimental Hematology in Milwaukee, there have probably been about 500 attempts to transplant bone marrow throughout the world.

Dr. Mortimer M. Bortin of Mount Sinai Hospital, Milwaukee, said the largest number of documented cases had been attempts to treat leukemia.

To date some of the most heartening successes have come in treating children born with serious defects in their own immunological defense systems.

Some of these children have been almost totally naked of any such defenses and therefore have been prey to terrible infection and early death from causes that would leave a normal person unmarked. In others the defects have been more circumscribed but still deadly.

Correction of these ordinarily fatal inborn defects has been possible only in about the past five years. The two classic cases were two little boys given marrow transplants in 1968; one by a team at the University of Minnesota led by Dr. Robert Good, the other by Dr. Fritz Bach and colleagues at the University of Wisconsin.

"For the first time, genetically determined inborn errors of metabolism have been fully corrected by a process of cellular engineering," Dr. Good said several years later in a report that covered these cases.

Now, more than four years after the transplants, the two boys are still healthy and are doing well in grade school; one in Connecticut, the other in upstate New York.

The transplant registry estimates there have been at least fourteen marrow grafts to correct immune deficiency from 1968 through the end of 1972 and eight of these are surviving more than a year after their operations. There have been eleven additional cases in which the grafts themselves did not take.

Among recent animal experiments that illustrate the ultimate potential promise of bone marrow transplantation are a series done in collaboration by a group at New York University led by Dr. Felix T. Rapaport and one at Mary Imogene Bassett Hospital in Cooperstown, N.Y., led by Dr. J. W. Ferrebee.

They have worked with a colony of beagle dogs maintained for many years at the hospital. Through careful analysis, the tissue types of these dogs have been worked out far more thoroughly than has been possible to date in man.

By choosing pairs that match perfectly—some littermates, others not—the scientists have achieved seventeen consecutive successful marrow transplants. Furthermore, once the bone marrow transplants were functioning, the animals also proved tolerant to kidney transplants from the same donors.

A long-range implication of this work is that someday a similar method might be used to make heart, kidney, or liver recipients permanently tolerant to their transplants by giving them bone marrow transplants from the prospective donor first. At present, of course, the life-and-death hazards of marrow transplantation in man rule out this strategy. If typing of human tissues ever reaches the refinement achieved with the beagles at Cooperstown, a whole new era in transplantation may result.

Experience to date with all kinds of transplants in man at many centers shows that lives can be saved even when scientific knowledge of the immunological problem is imperfect. But there is also evidence that the long-range results are best at those centers where the immunological barrier is taken most seriously.

Dr. Norman Shumway's heart transplant team at Stanford University, for example, is responsible for more than half of the heart transplant patients who survive today. Sir Michael F. A. Woodruff, of Edinburgh, an internationally known figure in transplantation and 1973 president of the Transplantation Society, remarked that he thought a large measure of the Stanford group's success could be attributed to their concern for the patient's immunological problems.

At the society's Fourth International Congress in San Francisco, some 500 transplant patients had a chance to meet and discuss common problems with the men and women who made their extended lives possible.

The final word at this unprecedented meeting was spoken by Sir Peter Medawar, the English scientist who won a Nobel Prize in 1960 for research that laid the basis for many of the advances that are bearing fruit today.

Looking out over the audience of scientists and beneficiaries of that science, he told them all that he had a feeling of "very great encouragement and renewed confidence that the goals of transplantation research are really worth striving for.

"It does seem amazing that we have come so far," he said, "but there is still a long way to go."

5

THE OLD AND
THE NEW

M EASLES is, beyond question, a virus infection. The virus has been identified, seen under the electron microscope, captured, tamed, and made into a vaccine that prevents the disease. Yet, when a person gets this unpleasant illness, it isn't really the virus that causes the pain and discomfort. For most of the symptoms of measles we have to blame the natural immunological counterattack by which the victim conquers his infection.

The typical child exposed to measles suffers no demonstrable ill effects at all for about ten days—during which time the virus is multiplying rapidly inside his body. A scientist who looks closely enough, using modern techniques, can find unmistakable evidence that the virus is present and multiplying, but the "patient" would find this hard to believe.

Then, abruptly, come the fever, rash, cough, itching, redness of the eyes, and swelling of the face. These symptoms may last three or four days. Then the fever, which may have risen above 104, and most of the other marks of the illness fade away almost as suddenly as they appeared. Thereafter, the victim of this virus is forever immune to it.

"It is clear that the disease which we have always called

measles is in fact an immune process that brings the real measles infection to an end," as a recent review of progress in immunology stated.

One of the main themes that runs through research in this field is that immunity is both good and bad—life-saving sometimes; life-threatening at others. It is both commonplace and mysterious. And the medical uses of immunity are at once among man's oldest and newest weapons against disease.

The immune reaction that brings a measles infection to a close is ordinarily good, albeit painful. But, as a few parents have discovered with horror every year, measles isn't always a harmless "common childhood disease." Sometimes, for reasons that are still obscure, it can lead to encephalitis—a dangerous inflammation of brain tissue that can permanently damage the mind and sometimes kill the patient. Only one case in every 1,200 or 1,500 develops this serious complication, but in pre-vaccine days, when every child was almost certain to get measles sooner or later, that still meant a large number of tragedies every year.

Within the past decade, the measles virus has also been linked to an even more deadly type of illness so uncommon that even its name is largely unknown except to specialists. In fact, it has been known by more than a half dozen different names because different doctors, discovering it at different times and places have each given it different names, not realizing that others had found and named it previously.

None of these names is easy to remember. The currently favored one is subacute sclerosing panencephalitis. It is usually called by the initials SSPE.

It is a rare disease of childhood but perhaps not quite as rare as had once been thought. More than 100 cases have been found in the United States alone, most of them in recent years. It is usually noticed first by the parents who gradually awaken to the frightening knowledge that their child's intellect is deteriorating. The next sign is strange periodic muscle spasms of the arms, legs, and trunk. The loss of mental and physical skills gets rapidly worse and worse. Usually the child dies within months. There is no cure; not even any useful treatment.

It used to be considered a rare hereditary defect. It is now known to be a bizarre outcome of virus infection. The virus? Measles.

The full story of how and why the deadly disease occurs is still to be told. The link to measles virus was first discovered around 1965 when doctors were surprised to find that victims of the disease had extraordinarily high levels of antibodies against measles in their blood. The levels got higher as the disease progressed. In 1969 the virus was actually recovered from brain tissue of patients who had died of the disease.

Somehow, the disease process causes damage to the brain tissues. The best guess at present is that there is something abnormal in the confrontation between the virus and the victim's immune defenses; possibly something abnormal in the defenses themselves.

All this makes it clear that there is a malevolent Mr. Hyde lurking within the immunological Dr. Jekyll who gives us so much help. The search for better understanding of that malevolence is one of the key concerns of modern research. We will return to it later. There is much to be learned about the beneficial side of the great defense system too, but parts of it are an old, old story. For immune processes gave doctors one of their first real weapons against illness, and, as we have said, physicians were manipulating the defense system centuries before they had any clear idea of what it was or, really, what they were doing.

Doctors in the orient had reputedly been immunizing people against smallpox long before Jenner's cowpox discovery. But they used material from human smallpox sores, choosing mild cases in the hope that the recipient's luck would be as good as that of the donor. Sometimes it worked and sometimes the patient died of smallpox.

Dr. Jenner found a safer way of doing the job. In doing so, he put immunology and virus research on a scientific basis a century before the first virus was discovered.

It is part of the colossal irony in man's long warfare against disease that this idea, old before Jenner's time, was yet so slowed by human ignorance, fear, and apathy that smallpox outbreaks still caused deaths in the United States in the 1930s. Only in the 1970s has mankind come close to eradicating the deadly virus from the whole world.

From Jenner's time onward, the most potent applications of immunology to human health have come through the use of vaccines. The common principle on which they all work is that of giving the individual a harmless exposure to a virus, bacterium, or other germ to stimulate the production of antibodies against it and thus render the person immune to the "wild" disease-causing type of the same germ.

Fundamentally there are two main ways of doing this. Jenner's method is the oldest and still the best. That is to find and use a "live," but harmless variant of the virus. This is exactly what the eighteenth century English physician did when he took material from the cowpox sores of a milkmaid to use in protecting another person against smallpox. Jenner's observation that milkmaids seldom if ever got smallpox led him to the brilliant thought that something in the cowpox infection—which seemed to give them a few sores and nothing else—must be protecting them against the far more dangerous smallpox infection.

Today doctors realize that the vaccinia and smallpox viruses are so closely related that immunity to one also confers immunity to the other. That same principle is the basis for the vaccines against polio, measles, rubella, mumps, yellow fever, and some other virus diseases. Bacteriologists have developed many laboratory tricks for finding or developing harmless strains of otherwise dangerous viruses. For example, they may grow viruses at unusual temperatures in the laboratory hoping to find a particular strain that prospers only in a temperature range that doesn't occur inside the human body.

A vaccine made from such a strain would sound the alarm for antibody production once it gets inside the human body, but the virus would not grow effectively and therefore would be eliminated without causing disease.

Live virus vaccines can be given either by injection or by mouth depending on the virus. In recent years thought has also been given to administering some vaccines into the nose by spray. This is considered a possibly effective route for vaccines against respiratory disease viruses. The rationale is that the antibodies most effective in preventing diseases of this type are secreted in the linings of the nasal and respiratory tract. An injected vaccine would lead primarily to production of antibodies in the blood stream and these would be less effective than the so-called local antibodies in preventing that particular infection.

The alternative to live virus vaccines is to use either a killed virus, or in the case of bacterial disease, antigen-rich extracts of those bacteria. The Salk vaccine that put polio on the road to public health oblivion, and the first measles vaccine, were both of the killed-virus type. The flu vaccines in use today, and some others, are of the killed-virus types. The killed-virus polio and measles vaccines have been replaced by live-virus alternatives because the latter tend to give more solid and durable immunity than the killed types. There are still some important diseases, however, for which the killed or inactivated type of vaccine is still used.

Whether the vaccine be inactivated or live, it generally

has to be given before the patient is exposed to the disease. It takes time for solid immunity to develop.

When there is no time, or when no vaccine against the disease exists, another strategy is sometimes used. This is passive immunization. In effect, the patient borrows antibodies from someone else by taking an injection of gamma globulin, the antibody-containing blood fraction. In some situations this protects against the disease so long as the borrowed antibodies continue to circulate in the blood, but it gives no lasting immunity. That last point, of course, is the reason for using a special gamma globulin in treating Rh negative mothers. Lasting immunity to the Rh blood factor is just what the doctor wants to prevent.

Except for the case of the Rh negative mother, all of the types of immunization used today must be regarded as fruits of "old fashioned" immunology. Technology and understanding have improved vastly, but philosophically it is still a replay of Dr. Jenner and cowpox. Nevertheless, the effects on public health have been incalculable.

The National Foundation, which was the chief sponsor of the war against polio, has estimated that 154,000 cases of the disease, including 12,500 deaths and 36,400 cases of severe paralysis were prevented by immunization in the first seven years after the Salk vaccine was introduced in 1954.

The savings have continued because polio, which sometimes hit 40,000 to 50,000 Americans a year before the vaccines were developed, is now a rare disease. A cluster of a few cases anywhere in the country is today termed an "outbreak" and is viewed with concern by public health officials who see such episodes as proof that the vaccine is not being used as widely as it should be.

Even discounting the factor of human health and well-being—which, after all, is the main point—modern vaccines can be defined as "cost effective" in cold-blooded dollars and cents terms.

The NIH immunology task force estimated that it may cost $5 million a year to support 100 scientists working in the fields of virus research, immunology, and related fields that give rise to vaccines. In contrast, it has been estimated that the vaccines in current use in this country save at least $1 billion a year in medical, hospital, and disability costs. It is hard to prove the accuracy of the estimates because they have to be calculated on something hypothetical—what might have happened if vaccines had not been developed. It seems unarguable, however, that the cost of developing vaccines has been repaid many times by the benefits they have given humanity. If no one can quite calculate their impact it is because vaccines have changed the world.

In a sense, the days of "easy" vaccine development may be past. Polio, tetanus, smallpox, diphtheria, whooping cough, measles, rubella, and mumps have all been conquered.

None of these victories seemed easy before the fact, although the technology is virtually commonplace today.

Influenza has at least been curtailed somewhat and protection is becoming available against some of the causes of deadly meningitis infections.

But all these victories and partial victories still leave a universe of disease. Experts in immunology think there are still huge areas where this field of science could make great progress.

For example, immunology might prove to be the ultimate best hope against malaria and other parasite diseases that remain the greatest public health problems in large areas of the world. A panel of the immunology task force said gamma globulin from immune adults has suppressed malaria infection in children and attempts at vaccination have been successful against the parasite that causes leishmaniasis, a common disease of the Middle East, Asia, and Africa. Obviously gamma globulin is not the answer to malaria any more than it was the answer to polio. There simply wouldn't be enough of it regardless of cost. But the demonstration shows that immunologic weapons can affect the disease. Perhaps other ways could be found to exploit these defenses more powerfully.

Closer to practical reality is the hope of vaccination against pneumococcus bacteria. While these germs don't account for all of the illness described as pneumonia, they are a major cause probably accounting for thousands of American deaths a year.

Research has already shown that a person can be immunized against a specific type of pneumococcus by a vaccine made of purified sugar-like substances called polysaccharides extracted from the outer capsules of the bacterial cells. A program, sponsored by the National Institute of Allergy and Infectious Diseases, is studying the practical usefulness of such vaccines including one product that would protect against six different pneumococcus types at once and another that would be effective against twelve.

Altogether there are eighty-two known types, but experts say that only twelve of these account for more than four fifths of the infections and three quarters of the deaths in adults. Eight types account for 70 percent of the infections in children. So, specialists believe vaccines can achieve much additional progress against the no longer fashionable, but still dangerous and prevalent bacterial pneumonias.

On theoretical grounds, and certainly from the standpoint of need, venereal disease ought to be a good subject for immunologic attack. Gonorrhea has been called the second most widespread infectious disease in the United States today; dwarfed only by the common cold. It is certainly the most widespread single reportable disease. There are far fewer cases of syphilis, but it too is alarmingly common and either out of control or in danger of becoming so, depending on one's point of view.

If vaccines could be developed and were widely used, these dangerous diseases could be conquered. Specialists say new advances in immunology could also help bring into being better means of diagnosis and treatment.

But for years study of the bacteriology and immunology of these diseases has been neglected. One of the main reasons for this neglect was probably the overconfidence of the early days of the antibiotic era. With pencillin and other drugs available, these diseases seemed to be all but conquered. Unfortunately, the conquest was never quite achieved. A substantial amount of new research would probably be needed to make vaccines possible against gonorrhea and syphilis. Unfortunately, there is much more at stake here than the science. Venereal disease is no longer considered unspeakable and unmentionable as it was just a few decades ago, but that doesn't mean that all of the moral stigma has been lifted. Reseach to pursue the vaccine goal has clearly been impeded by the social implications.

There are some who would still argue that vaccination against either of these diseases would represent a license for promiscuity and should therefore be taboo no matter how much suffering the vaccines could prevent. While disease control by moral stricture certainly has not worked in the past, there are still some vocal zealots to argue that this is the only way.

Imagine the oratory that might blossom forth in Congress if anyone proposed a national crusade against venereal disease based on a goal as unspiritual as vaccination.

Like the current crusade against cancer, an effort against venereal disease would take substantial amounts of money, manpower, and research. Yet, while congressmen and the president found it impossible to be "against" cancer research, they might find it hazardous to be "for" a venereal vaccine crusade. So the one area of research most likely to find a permanent answer to these horrible diseases is likely to remain only modestly funded and the hope of conquest will remain largely theoretical.

Strangely enough, the common cold seems no more likely than venereal disease to be conquered by vaccination. The reasons are entirely different.

The current golden age of virus hunting has nowhere been more successful than in finding viruses that cause colds. The search for the agents of the sneezes and sniffles has centered on a group called the rhinoviruses—rhino being derived from the Greek word for nose. Starting in about 1956, scientists have been plagued by an embarrassment of riches in their search. They have found not one, nor several, but a whole army of different rhinoviruses. The total stands now at about 100. It is possible to produce antibodies and, presumably, immunity against any of them.

The trouble is that antibodies against one give no substantial protection against the others and a combined vaccine against 100 different virus types is far beyond the present capabilities of vaccine-makers. To complicate the problem, rhinoviruses are difficult to deal with in the laboratory. Many of them can be grown only in human embryonic tissue. There are no simple tools by which epidemiologists can find them efficiently and study their distribution in man.

At best, the average American, intent on avoiding next winter's colds, would have to take 100 different shots. These simply aren't available, however, and it is probably just as well that they aren't.

In a recent summary report, Dr. George B. Mackaness,

director of the Trudeau Institute at Saranac Lake, N.Y., said the rhinoviruses evidently cause only about 25 percent of common colds; primarily those that come in fall and winter. Another group of viruses—called coronoviruses—has been discovered to cause about eight percent of winter and spring colds. At least two or three coronovirus types have been identified and there is no assurance that some others don't exist as well.

Perhaps an additional 10 percent of the illnesses the victims call colds are caused by influenza and parainfluenza viruses. That still leaves more than half of all common colds unaccounted for. The causes are unknown and cures must still be left to the individual's natural defenses. The cold remedies, for which Americans spend millions of dollars every year, give psychological comfort and perhaps some relief of some symptoms. But that is all.

Vaccines have probably had more impact on human well-being than any other human health measures except sanitation and insect control. The most effective vaccines have been those against "conventional" virus infections such as polio, mumps, measles, and smallpox in which the infection becomes quickly and painfully obvious. It hardly takes a doctor more than a few minutes to diagnose a case of measles when he sees a child with the appropriate spots, fever, and other symptoms. There are no great difficulties in smallpox either, although most American doctors have never actually seen a case.

But, today much research attention is being turned toward

an entirely different situation—the case of the so-called "slow virus infection." These infections are the province of the "new" immunology and the "new" virology. The action of the virus is slow but inexorable, subtle but finally devastating. The period of latency, in which the virus particles are present but undetected, is sometimes measured in years rather than days or a very few weeks.

These bizarre infections are interesting to scientists because some of them are so out of the ordinary as to suggest an entirely new class of infectious particles in the "sea of microorganisms" in which the world is bathed. To doctors and public health workers the slow infections are also more than moderately interesting. The behavior of these virus infections in animals and, to some extent, in man, is reminiscent of some important and totally puzzling human diseases of the nervous system. The most widely known of these is multiple sclerosis.

In fact, the educated guessing among some scientists close to the problem is that multiple sclerosis will prove to be a slow virus infection. This idea has been gaining ground for several years but, so far, has been impossible to prove. To a great extent the burden of proof will rest on immunology. Certainly if this crippling and ultimately fatal illness does prove to be a virus disease it will be up to the immunologists, more than any other discipline, to figure out how to deal with it.

The aberrant virus diseases that have been discovered in recent years are far different from anything recognized in the past. Furthermore, not all of these infections are alike. So far the most common trend is that those documented to date all seem to affect the nervous system. This is true, for example of the rare disease called SSPE in which the victim loses control over both body and mind over a period of months and then dies.

In its effects on brain and central nervous system, SSPE resembles the strange disease called kuru which, in many ways, is the classic of its kind. But there are also marked differences between the two. SSPE appears to be closely related to the measles virus and its victims have extraordinarily high levels of antimeasles antibody before they die.

In kuru, on the other hand, scientists have not been able to find antibodies against anything that could be the cause of the fatal illness.

In fact, kuru is certainly one of the most mysterious and exotic human diseases ever discovered. The man mainly responsible for our present knowledge of it is Dr. D. Carleton Gajdusek, of the National Institute of Neurological Diseases and Stroke.

In the mid-1950s he was among the first Western doctors to study the disease in the wild highlands of New Guinea, the only place on earth where it is known to exist. Its only known victims are natives called the Fore people and some others who have intermarried with them. They aren't exactly a tribe, but share similarities of language throughout a population of about 12,000. They all live in a small region in the easternmost part of inland New Guinea.

In the 1950s it looked as though they all might be doomed by kuru. The illness was always fatal and it had reached epidemic proportions in some of the villages. Most of the victims were women and children. The Fore people might die out entirely if the trend continued.

On the average, the illness lasted about a year or less. The victim first became aware of it as an unsteadiness in gait, sometimes preceded by headaches and pains in the limbs. Loss of coordination and tremors of the head and limbs, often aggravated by cold, made up the next phase. By that time the victim knew that she was going to die.

In the Fore language, the word kuru means to shake or shiver from cold or fear.

In later stages, the victims suffered slurred speech, inability to control the eyes and limbs and a mental deterioration the doctors describe as mild dementia. By the time the patients actually died they were emaciated, mute, and totally helpless.

The Fore people are extremely primitive and isolated. Although they live on an island, most of them had never seen the sea nor traveled more than a few miles from the place they were born. Their language didn't even have a word for ocean. They also seemed to have no concept of sanitation. One of the first thoughts of those who studied the epidemic was that it might be caused by a virus, but this was abandoned because there was no evidence to support it. A more likely possibility seemed to be that it was a genetic disease, although kuru wasn't easy to explain in those terms either.

From the traditions of the villagers, it seemed that kuru had probably first appeared in one village about forty or fifty years ago and then spread gradually throughout the population. It couldn't have been much longer than that, because, at the rate it was killing people, there wouldn't have been any Fore people left. During the years they worked in New Guinea, Dr. Gajdusek and his colleagues collected records of more than 1,400 cases of the disease.

For years, kuru didn't seem to make any scientific sense. It was hard to explain in terms of heredity, but even more difficult if one tried to find some causative poison in the diet. Infection by an unknown virus was a tempting theory, but the doctors could find no characteristic antibodies, no abnormalities in the blood or lymph system; nothing. Furthermore, it didn't seem to be transmissible from person to person even under conditions of extreme close contact and incredibly lacking sanitation.

The solution to the mystery came from animal experiments by Dr. Gajdusek and his colleagues in the United States and close observation of the Fore people in their villages in New Guinea.

It did prove to be a virus disease, although a most unusual one. The final proof of this came when scientists injected filtered material from the brains of the victims into eight chimpanzees in the laboratory. After months in which nothing seemed to be happening, the animals developed symptoms just like those of kuru. Material from their brains proved capable of passing the disease to still other primates.

In a recent report Dr. Peter W. Lampert, University of California, San Diego, Dr. Gajdusek, and Dr. Clarence J.

Gibbs, Jr., one of Dr. Gajdusek's principal co-workers at the NIH, said the fatal virus can now be transmitted to a wide variety of animals. It seems to do its damage exclusively in brain and nerve tissue.

Since the material can still cause disease after passage through a filter of extremely small pore size, it is clearly a virus; but it must be injected to cause the disease. How was it transmitted among the Fore people, who had never seen a hypodermic needle before Western doctors arrived?

The answer proved to be one of the most bizarre parts of the whole story.

The Fore people were cannibals. As they saw life, cannibalism was not something you did to your enemies, but a special mark of affection for friends and relatives who had just died. At elaborate funeral ceremonies, the women of the tribe removed the brain of the dead person and the mourners shared in eating it. Through this custom kuru passed among them.

How kuru got started in the first place will probably never be known. Perhaps it was a mutant virus that struck one member of a village and then was passed on to the next generation and from person to person and village to village because of the fateful funeral custom. According to Dr. Gajdusek and his colleagues, the Fore people believe their affliction began roughly forty to fifty years ago. Perhaps significantly, their strange funeral feast of the dead is believed to have started at just about the same time.

Evidently the disease was not spread simply by eating the brain tissue of the infected victim. Had that been the case, the epidemic would have spread even faster than it did.

In the animal experiments that proved kuru to be a virus disease, the malady could be passed on only by injecting extracts of the brain tissue, not by feeding it. Evidently that was also how it was passed from person to person in the Fore villages.

It wasn't intentional, but that seems to have been what happened. The women who removed the brains for the ceremonial feast, Dr. Gajdusek says, did the job with razor sharp bamboo slivers. From time to time they tested the sharpness of their instruments by pricking themselves in the forearms—and unknowingly must have given themselves small injections of kuru virus as they did so. Children in the villages also helped prepare for the feasts. They may have gotten the virus through the usual cuts and scrapes and other small wounds of childhood.

The disease was untreatable and incurable. It might well have destroyed the entire people. But about the same time that Western doctors and scientists began to study the Fore villages, other harbingers of civilization were becoming entrenched too. A police patrol post was set up at one of the villages in 1951. Missionaries became established there in 1953. Somehow, the Fore people were persuaded to find ways of honoring their dead other than eating them. Although the coincidence was only recognized later, when the ritual cannibalism stopped the disease stopped gaining ground and soon began to decline.

The virus that causes kuru is still a major puzzle to

virologists and immunologists alike. It is remarkably re-sistant to heat, cold, and the chemicals that normally break down DNA and RNA, the active materials in the core of all known viruses. When scientists look for kuru virus par-ticles under the electron microscope all they have been able to see is what looks like fragments of cell membrane. In a recent report on this and other slow virus diseases, Drs. Gajdusek and Gibbs mention the possibility that kuru may be caused by a hitherto unknown type of infectious sub-stance which might be little more than a self-replicating membrane fragment free of either DNA or RNA. They also note, however, that the kuru virus may prove to be simply a small conventional virus with some most unconventional properties.

All this is fascinating to virologists and puzzling to im-munologists who find it hard to understand why so potent and destructive an agent seems to leave no immunologic traces of its presence.

The interest is heightened by this fact: bizarre as it is, kuru is not the only virus disease of its kind. In a survey report, Drs. Lampert, Gibbs, and Gajdusek said it is one of four known slow virus diseases close enough in their similarities to be considered a single disease class. Two of these are animal diseases; scrapie, a long-known fatal affliction of sheep, and a disease of ranch-bred mink called transmissible mink encephalopathy.

The other two are kuru, known only in one restricted region of New Guinea; and a rare, but more widely dis-tributed fatal illness called Creutzfeldt-Jakob disease. It is named after two doctors who, independently, found cases of the same disease in different places but at about the same time—roughly fifty years ago, which by coincidence is about the time the Fore people estimate that kuru began among them.

Creutzfeldt-Jakob disease has been found in only a relatively few humans, but they have been scattered; some cases having been found in Europe, others in Canada and the United States.

All four of the diseases, two in animals, two in man, are fatal, progressive illnesses that involve destruction of tissues in the brain and central nervous system. All of them have proved to be transmissible to other animals by injection. They all appear to be caused by viruses, but the behavior of these viruses is extraordinary—from their long latent periods of months or more than a year in their victims, to their resistance to things that destroy most viruses.

Unlike multiple sclerosis, which some scientists believe is also the result of a slow virus infection, these four diseases do not eat away the myelin sheaths that insulate the nerve fibers.

Except, fortunately, for their rarity these strange slow-acting virus diseases fit the bill perfectly for one of the classic themes of science fiction. This is the theme of the human race being threatened by a mysterious infection—its cause undetectable, its effects beyond the powers of medicine to cure or prevent.

Perhaps no super germ of that sort could exist. Certainly the rarity of kuru and Creutzfeldt-Jakob disease suggest that some natural defenses must be protecting the bulk of humanity and animal species in general against that kind of deadly infection.

But such rare and deadly virus diseases do point up the importance of learning more about how the body's natural defenses work—and how they sometimes fail or misbehave. Examples ranging from measles—once among the most common of the common infections of man—to kuru—unknown beyond one group of people living in one of the most isolated places on earth—show how important this understanding can be.

The immunological system can protect. It can cure. Inexplicably it can seemingly keep hands off, as in kuru and to some extent leprosy as well as other diseases. Clearly, it can also be the source of the trouble itself, but that is the next part of the story.

6

THE MANY-EDGED
SWORD

I was a little thing, presumably harmless; a few drops of red pigment from guinea pig blood injected into the skin. Yet, in just 16 minutes the healthy young woman who received it was dead. She was a volunteer in a medical experiment thought to be entirely safe, but her body reacted violently. Within minutes she complained of headache and began to wheeze. Her skin turned blue. Despite everything doctors could do for her in those remaining few minutes, she died.

The cause was an immunologic reaction gone wild. The woman's internal defense system had reacted too powerfully too soon to an intrusion of something foreign.

That reaction, called anaphylactic shock, kills an estimated 30 persons a year from such trivial causes as bee stings; and kills a substantially larger number who react violently to antibiotics such as penicillin.

This is the bad side of the complex defense system that helps protect humans from germs and parasites and probably cancer; a defense almost as old as life itself, without which we would all die. Not surprisingly, this immunological bulwark has its own derangements. It is potent and life-

113

preserving, but its destructive power can also work against the body's best interests.

That happens not only in rare emergencies like anaphylactic shock, but also in common allergies that afflict an estimated 31 million Americans. The immunologic system is probably an important factor in such widespread and debilitating illnesses as rheumatoid arthritis, multiple sclerosis, some forms of kidney disease and anemia, and in many other conditions with less familiar names.

Some scientists believe immune processes are at work, harmfully, in atherosclerosis—that form of hardening of the arteries which lies at the root of heart disease and is the number one killer of Americans. Some even suspect that the process of aging itself is a partially immunological "disease."

All these lines of evidence and conjecture are the subject of intense study today. The good and bad effects of the immune defenses seem to turn up almost everywhere. Their mechanisms seem to be woven through almost every aspect of the life process. This becomes more and more apparent as research reveals more of the detailed mechanisms through which the defenses function; and more of the effects these same mechanisms bring about.

When the strange case of the reaction to guinea pig blood went into the files of Harvard Medical School's Department of Legal Medicine a few decades ago, anaphylaxis was already an old story. But only its effects and the broad outline of its causes were clear.

Even today, no one knows exactly what brings on these

rare tragedies that have been called "allergic sudden death." Scientists do know the specific class of substances within the body that starts the reaction. They have even been able to trace some of the chemical events that lead to disaster. This is of widespread importance.

Although the number of people endangered each year by anaphylaxis is extremely small, the number of things capable of inciting such an attack is large. Usually, the fatal cases result from injection of the material to which the victim is hypersensitive, but sometimes the sensitivity is so razor sharp that even things taken by mouth can bring on a life-threatening attack.

Attacks have been brought on by injected drugs including penicillin, the local anesthetic procaine, the antituberculosis drug PAS, vaccines, gamma globulin, insulin, blood transfusion, and even some food products. Anaphylaxis can kill because the victim's breathing becomes obstructed by swelling in the larynx or by spasm of the bronchial passages. It can also kill either from derangement of heart rhythm or because of sudden fall in blood pressure. The victim is likely to be dead within a half hour of the event that triggers the attack, often less.

If the patient is lucky enough to be near a hospital or doctor's office he can usually be saved. Depending on the individual case, he may need airways restored, heart rhythm corrected, or a shot of epinephrine. If the crisis occurs far from help, there is little that can be done in time. As one expert put it, the best treatment is prevention.

Part of the importance of understanding these tragedies

lies in this fact: the same aspect of immunologic defense that can lead to anaphylaxis on rare occasions, leads much more commonly to the allergies that affect millions.

These include a whole host of afflictions from trivial to disabling caused by almost anything imaginable—food, pollen, house dust, drug, cosmetic, industrial chemical, poison ivy.

In fact, some real damage is probably done by allergies that don't actually exist. It is estimated that five percent of Americans are allergic to one or another drug—but that three times that many *think* they have a drug-allergy problem. Some in that latter group may be avoiding drugs that they really need for fear of allergies they really don't have.

For that reason as well as all the other obvious ones, physicians, chemists, immunologists, and many others are trying to learn more about the bad side of immunology.

An important key to it is a class of antibodies called Immunoglobulin E—IgE, for short. The special functions of these antibodies were discovered just a few years ago by a husband and wife team now at Johns Hopkins University, but then at the Children's Asthma Research Institute and Hospital in Denver. They are Dr. Kimishige Ishizaka and his wife, Dr. Teruko Ishizaka.

Although antibodies are commonly called defensive proteins, these sometimes act more like vandals.

To recapitulate some of the fundamentals: antibodies circulate in the blood and react with foreign material to which the body has been sensitized. Five main types have been discovered. The three best known are Immunoglobulin G, which defends mainly against invading bacteria, other germs, and foreign proteins; A, which is secreted in the nose, digestive tract, and other places to give local protection against invasion; and M, which is usually the first to be formed against an invader. The role of immunoglobulin D is yet to be discovered.

The Ishizakas' discovery that the IgE class is a factor in allergic reactions is considered a milestone in modern medical research.

One of the key characteristics of antibodies in general is their incredible specificity. An antibody designed to react with polio virus type 2, for example, will not respond to type 1 or 3 even though the differences between the three are unimaginably small.

That specificity explains much of their importance in the immunological defense apparatus. They are like sentries able to tell friend from foe and call the troops into action.

The way IgE performs that latter function is one of the most important discoveries concerning it. These antibodies seem to function through a lock-and-key matching between one end of the antibody and the offending foreign substance and another lock-and-key match between the other end of the antibody molecule and a body cell called a mast cell.

Somehow, when this three-way link is established in a sensitized person, the mast cell goes into action. It squirts out histamine and another chemical known as the slow reacting substance—which works in seconds rather than the fraction of a second in which histamine exerts its effects—and something called a chemotactic factor, which attracts certain white blood cells called eosinophils.

Altogether these chemical warfare agents of the body are capable of producing all the effects that cause woe to the allergy patient—the swollen membranes, runny nose, watery eyes, and difficulty in breathing.

By studying slices of human tissue in the laboratory, doctors have found that this constellation of chemicals released from mast cells can make smooth muscles, such as those of the bronchial tubes, contract; make blood vessels a little leaky so that fluids escape from them. The attraction of the eosinophils also seems to be a part of the process, but just what they do once on the scene is not yet clearly known.

Dr. K. Frank Austen of Robert B. Brigham Hospital and Harvard Medical School in Boston has been among the pioneers in these studies of the so-called "mediators" of the allergic and inflammatory responses and the systems through which they act.

"There has been tremendous progress in our understanding of these effector systems," he said during a recent interview. The next step is to identify the diseases in which the systems are abnormal because this could have major implications for understanding cause and improving treatment.

For example, he said, the discoveries in recent years help explain why antihistamine drugs are only partially effective in coping with allergic conditions. They deal with one of the mediators, not the others.

To some research workers this suggests that an effective way of dealing with allergy problems in a patient might be through drugs that would reduce the tendency of mast cells, and others acted upon by IgE, to release powerful chemicals.

In a recent scientific report Dr. Kimishige Ishizaka showed evidence from experiments in rabbits suggesting another approach.

He said it appears that a specific subclass of immunologically active white blood cells is responsible for the formation of the IgE antibodies.

By inactivating these cells alone, while leaving intact others responsible for other groups of antibodies, allergic reactivity might be damped down. The broader implication is that each type of antibody is controlled by its own subpopulation of immunologically active cells and might be subject to control through them.

The activities of IgE and the other agents of allergic reactivity constitute only one facet of the huge and complex panorama of immunological effects that can do either harm or good.

Indeed, as Dr. John R. David, of Robert Brigham Hospital, points out, the immune mechanisms are the same whether the person involved finds the effects good or bad. If the reactions are helpful—resistance to disease-causing germs, or destruction of cancer cells, for example—the effect is usually described as "immunity."

When the same mechanisms produce injury to a person's own tissues, one usually refers to the condition as "hypersensitivity." But the distinction between the two is really largely in the eye of the beholder, depending on whether he considers the effect good or bad.

The mechanisms themselves are incredibly complex, full of redundancies, separate systems that produce similar end-results, cooperative activities between cells of different kinds; and a multitude of things that mediate, enhance, and sometimes turn off a sequence of immunologic events.

For example, there are the two major classes of immunologic defense: humoral immunity involving circulating antibodies and all the systems and substances that act with them; and cellular immunity with an overlapping, but in some ways distinct set of functions.

The white blood cells called T lymphocytes are a major factor in the cellular system. They, too, have a complex set of mediators, first described only about six years ago and still not completely understood.

As Dr. David describes these, there appear to be at least four. They include a migration inhibitory factor, which keeps scavenger cells called macrophages at the spot where defense against invasion must be mounted and, more important, heightens the activity and aggressiveness of the macrophages.

There is also a chemotactic factor, which brings defensively active white cells to the scene; a toxic product capable of killing cells; another factor that may make the cells useful in defense multiply. There may also be an antiviral substance.

Existence of all of these is indicated by experiments in the test tube. The question still to be answered is whether or not they actually function according to this scenario in man. If they do, these functions, both specific and generalized, would help greatly in explaining why the immunological system is so strong in defense and so destructive when its powers are turned against its own body.

One of the key ingredients in the humoral defense system is an extraordinarily complex set of substances called the complement system. It was originally thought to be a single substance that served to complete the actions of antibodies.

It is now known to consist of at least nine major proteins and several other lesser ones all activated in sequence after being triggered by the antibodies that react with bacteria, viruses, or tissues that the antibodies recognize as foreign. It has a wide variety of functions, ranging from effects on blood coagulation to producing changes in the surfaces of bacteria to make them more easily attacked and engulfed by scavenger cells.

Dr. Hans J. Muller-Eberhard, of Scripps Clinic and Research Foundation, La Jolla, Calif., one of the major figures in research on the system, says most of the present knowledge concerning it was unforeseen as recently as ten years ago.

121

The available evidence shows that, for all its complexity, the complement system is no more complicated than the body's needs for it require.

The requirements are basically that it respond to the recognition of a foreign invader by antibodies, that it mobilize and act destructively against the invader, and that it avoid acting on false clues or insufficient evidence. Basically the complement system seems designed to affect cell membranes, and this gives it a key role in defending the body.

Even so, the complement system can be a factor in human disease when one or another of its components is missing—particularly when the absent item is one of the control factors designed to hold the destructive activity in check.

Some of the experts on complement believe this system developed even before immunological defenses arose in the course of evolution. In early forms of life, all-out attack was the answer to any threat. Only later was complement harnessed, so to speak, by the immunologic defense system, thus giving the former a degree of specificity it probably lacked originally.

Suggestive of this early origin is the fact that creatures as primitive as starfish, although lacking antibodies, do have a variant of the complement system called the "alternate pathway." This argues that something akin to complement must have been protecting the integrity of ancient creatures that were experimenting with life's possibilities in the early seas hundreds of millions of years ago.

Today, as is true of other portions of the defense system, complement is also thought to be a factor in some diseases when circumstances conspire to turn it loose in the wrong way.

Several years ago, scientists in the United States and Sweden found, almost simultaneously, that rheumatoid arthritis patients had marked abnormalities of the complement system detectable in the fluid of their affected joints. This has been studied by many laboratories here and abroad and is widely believed to be true.

Much earlier, scientists noted something that has been named rheumatoid factor in the serum of the rheumatoid arthritis patient. This has proved to be a complex of two different antibodies, one presumably directed at whatever it may be that originally sparked the arthritic condition and the other against that first antibody.

Dr. Austen notes that this may be a self-perpetuating effect, persisting even after the original inciting agent, whatever it is, has disappeared. The effect may persist because the body is making antibodies against one of its own products.

He believes rheumatoid arthritis may well be a good example of an acquired immune complex disease in which the major mechanism of tissue injury is the involvement of the classic complement system.

The implication is that new ways of treating this difficult disease might be forthcoming if scientists could discover ways of turning off the self-destructive, self-pepetuating immunologic event.

Conceivably, important progress along these lines could be made even before research workers find an answer to the key question of the whole intricate puzzle: what is the "X factor" that starts the whole process in the first place?

Indeed, possibilities such as this are among the things that evoke so much interest in the immunologic aspects of disease. The system has so many complexities that it seems to offer many potential points of intervention at which some carefully designed treatment could turn off the process that produces the damage.

In theory, this kind of intervention would also have the advantage of attacking the disease problem specifically with a minimum of those side-effects that accompany more generalized forms of treatment.

In an interview Dr. Hugh O. McDevitt, of Stanford University, one of the major figures in current immunology research, predicted that the next ten years would see vast advances in man's ability to interfere with the immunological processes that lead to allergic and inflammatory disease.

In contrast, some of the "miracle medicines" of the recent past are thought now to be relatively crude. One scientist in the Midwest described early efforts to use cortisone-type drugs against rheumatoid diseases as akin to "hunting pheasants with napalm."

The anti-inflammatory effect was certainly achieved, but often at great cost in side-effects. These drugs are still widely used, and are probably indispensable but doctors tend to be more and more sparing in their use.

The Many-Edged Sword

On the other hand, at least one treatment still considered useful in some rheumatoid arthritis patients came into the picture years ago through major misconceptions.

Dr. J. Sydney Stillman, 1971–72 president of the American Rheumatism Association, said the use of gold salts became popular several decades ago because of two basic mistakes: rheumatoid arthritis was thought to be related to tuberculosis and gold was thought to be useful against that infectious disease. Both proved to be wrong, but, for reasons still obscure, gold salts do seem to help some arthritis patients.

Of particular interest to specialists in immunology are diseases that have been classified loosely as "autoimmune," meaning that in whole or in part they result from damage done when the defense system turns against the body's own tissues.

There is a recent trend, some experts in this field say, to a change in definition to shift the emphasis to immunologically self-inflicted injury.

This, said Dr. Philip Y. Paterson, who is Samuel J. Sackett Professor of Medicine and Microbiology at Northwestern University, broadens the definition to include reactions that initially are against something foreign, but which damage native tissues as well. This would probably include such widespread diseases as rheumatoid arthritis and several important forms of anemia.

Dr. Paterson, who headed the panel of autoimmune disease of the task force on immunology organized by the National Institute of Allergy and Infectious Diseases, believes that shift in emphasis may be of far-ranging importance.

Diseases in which at least some of the damage appears to be done by the immune response include some of the most widespread and important afflictions of mankind.

As some scientists see the situation today, several important lines of study are beginning to converge: immunologic damage, key afflictions of mankind such as heart disease, cancer, and arthritis, and even that universal affliction of all mammals—the process of growing old.

For years, experts in autoimmune disease used to think mainly in terms of injury directed by the body against its own native cells. The newer thought that the inciting agent may come from the outside, broadens the concept hugely. It also brings viruses into the picture more solidly than ever before.

These tiny, malevolent particles have haunted many areas of chronic disease research for decades. They have been prime suspects in cancer, multiple sclerosis, and even rheumatoid arthritis to name just a few.

One scientist suggested wryly a few years ago that perhaps there ought to be an international research congress devoted to cancer, arthritis, heart and kidney ailments, mental illness, aging, "and other virus-caused diseases."

Today that seems a little less like a joke than it did originally.

Viruses can persist in the body for long periods of time,

producing effects that can be either subtle or devastating. The mysterious slow virus infections of man and animals demonstrate that.

There are several ways in which virus infection might set the stage for autoimmune disease. If viruses persist in cells of the body for long periods, passing from one generation of cells to the next repeatedly, the cells might become subtly altered. These alterations might be enough to make the immune defenses detect them as foreign. This could lead to a damaging immune reaction to those body tissues involved.

Some scientists think it more likely that the immune response called forth by the virus itself might cause injury to cells and tissues of the body. This might happen simply because the coexistence of viruses and cells is so close and intimate that damage would be unavoidable. It is difficult enough to shoot an apple off the top of a person's head without doing any harm. It would be well nigh impossible if the person were actually eating the apple at the time.

There is a third possible mechanism of injury in autoimmune disease that is much better documented than the others. This is damage arising from virus-antibody complexes. One of the prime functions of antibody is to combine with its target. In a persistent virus infection it may be that viral fragments and antibodies against them become glued together so to speak and circulate in the blood stream. Whenever such antigen-antibody complexes lodge in tissues their presence might call forth a whole barrage of inflammatory and injurious effects. It has been shown, for example, that some forms of kidney disease result from the disastrous effects of antigen-antibody complexes getting lodged in the small filter structures known as glomeruli.

Similarly, complexes that get lodged in brain tissue could bring disaster to that organ too. If the virus infection was widespread throughout the body, or if the circulating complexes became lodged in many places, the immunological injury would be widespread—in short, a systemic disease. These descriptions define what is now being called immune complex disease. There are important illnesses of man that seem to fit them perfectly. Among the possibilities are glomerulonephritis, a devastating kidney disease, and systemic lupus erythematosus, which can evoke symptoms of arthritis, skin rashes, fever, and which can be fatal when the kidneys or central nervous system become involved. Rheumatoid arthritis also fits the description. The so-called rheumatoid factor in the blood that is characteristic of this disease has proved to be antibody against the patient's own immunoglobulins. In other words, it is antibody against antibodies. Although rheumatoid arthritis does not ordinarily kill its victims, it can disable them sporadically over periods of many years. Between two and three million Americans are believed to be afflicted with it.

In all of these diseases, the role of immunology is becoming more and more apparent. Experts estimate, for example, that in at least nine tenths of glomerulonephritis cases the damage probably results from immune complexes getting trapped in the glomeruli. Still mysterious is what causes the complexes to form in the first place. This is where viruses come under suspicion.

If a virus could be identified as the original source of antigen that started the whole process, specialists would be much further along in understanding such a disease.

All this is of much more than theoretical interest. Immune complexes seem to form and persist only when the conditions are just right. Something as simple as a shift in the ratio of antigen to antibody might stop them. If so, why couldn't doctors force such a shift deliberately?

The tempting payoff for identifying specific antigens in immune complex disease, said a panel of the NIH immunology task force, is the possibility of manipulating the pathogenic response either up or down and thereby terminating the formation of circulating complexes.

Broadly speaking, this kind of ploy typifies the dream in the eye of immunologists today. They want to design treatment which would get at the core of the disease process. In all of these diseases, today's methods of treatment concentrate instead on fighting the symptoms. The underlying process that causes them is still beyond reach. The hope of immunology in all of these situations is to bring the basic disease process finally within their grasp.

Perhaps that possibility might someday extend to the greatest killer and crippler of all—diseases of the heart and circulatory system. Certainly immunologic factors are at work in rheumatic heart disease. There are some who think they may also be involved in more common afflictions of heart, blood vessels, and blood.

In some types of acquired anemia, doctors have found antibodies that become attached to the type of blood cell involved in the illness. Although the origin of the antibody is often unknown, the effects of its presence are clear. The body's scavenger system tends to remove the antibody-coated cells from circulation even if the antibody hasn't damaged the cell.

Immune processes may even have a bearing on the central process of atherosclerosis itself—the process that underlies most disease of heart and blood vessels. The blood substances called platelets tend to aggregate and cause blood coagulation when they become coated by antibody or by immune complexes. In this way immunologic damage may, conceivably, be a factor in the laying down of atherosclerotic plaques. It is these plaques that damage the arteries and set up the conditions for the most common forms of heart trouble.

Altogether, a case can be made for implicating the immunologic system—either as hero or villain—in most of the major health problems of mankind. Some research workers even see a role for the system in the health problem that finally usurps all others—the problem of growing old. Studies in man and mouse have shown that a normal individual peaks during adolescence in his ability to make antibodies when stimulated by a foreign antigen. After adolescence it is all downhill.

In the aged, cellular immunity has also fallen far below the levels of youth. Judging from the rising incidence of cancer in older age groups it could be guessed that the immunological surveillance system becomes jaded.

Meanwhile, autoimmune processes seem to become more frequent. It is almost as though the body finally wearies of the self-nonself argument it has been carrying on with its environment for a lifetime.

The truth is probably more prosaic and far more complex than that, but links between the immunologic system and the effects of aging turn up everywhere. Even some forms of the protein substance amyloid, which accumulates in aging tissues, including those of the brain, apparently consist mainly of abnormal light chains of immunoglobulin molecules. This could suggest that there is an immunologic factor even in senility.

Zealots in immunology, like their counterparts in other fields, tend to see their own specialty as the ultimate key to everything. This may call for the immune response of healthy skepticism. Nevertheless, it is certainly true that immunology has become an all but universal tool of research; that its investigations impinge on an ever-broadening range of health matters; and that it has opened vistas for the understanding of life that extend almost from the origin of animals to the final effects of old age on man.

Specialists in immunology expect their field to become more and more a central issue in the protection of human health in the years and decades immediately before us. Being so fundamental as a science and so precise as a tool, immunology seems to offer a whole new universe of possibilities for broadening human knowledge and for lifting the burden of illness from mankind.

GLOSSARY

Adjuvant—A substance that will enhance the immune response to an antigen when injected with the antigen.

Allergy—Abnormally heightened reactivity to an antigen. The term is usually used synonymously with immediate hypersensitivity; that is, hypersensitivity caused by antibodies of the gamma E class.

Anaphylaxis—A violent form of immediate hypersensitivity that can occur when a person already sensitive to a particular antigen is exposed to it.

Antibodies—Proteins in the blood that can combine with specific antigens. Antibodies are immunoglobulins.

Antigen—Anything that provokes a specific immune response in an individual; in short, anything that provokes an antibody response.

Asthma—A disease characterized by attacks of wheezing, difficulty in breathing, and over-inflation of the lungs. Some forms of asthma are produced by acute hypersensitivity reactions to antigens such as those of pollen.

Auto-antibody—An antibody capable of reacting with antigens native to the individual.

Auto-immune disease—Disease produced by self-inflicted immunological injury.

B cell—Also called a B lymphocyte, these are cells derived from progenitors in the bone marrow. The B cells, in turn, are progenitors of antibody-forming cells.

Bacillus Calmette-Guerin (BCG)—A special strain of tuberculosis bacteria used as a vaccine against that disease and also being used now in efforts to enhance a cancer patient's immune response to cancer tissue.

Blood Groups—Different types of blood distinguishable immunologically from each other because they have different characteristic antigens on the surface of the red blood cells. The most important blood groups in man are the ABO system, so-called because its main types have been designated A, B, and O.

Bone Marrow—Blood-forming tissue located in the cavities of the bones.

Cell-mediated immunity—Immune reactions mediated by T-cells rather than by antibodies.

Complement—A complex series of proteins in the blood serum which are activated by the reactions between antibodies and antigens.

Gamma globulin—The portion of blood serum that includes immunoglobulins and, therefore, antibodies.

GVH—Graft versus host disease; a dangerous condition that can result from injection in one person of immunologically active cells from a genetically dissimilar individual. It is a major problem in bone marrow transplantation.

Immunoglobulins—Those proteins in the blood that have antibody activity.

Leukocytes—White blood cells including lymphocytes.

Lymph nodes—Small organs distributed widely throughout the body which serve as filters through which foreign materials that get into the circulation must pass and come into close contact with lymphocytes.

Lymphocytes—Immunologically active cells such as B-cells and T-cells present in lymph nodes, spleen, and blood.

Macrophages—Scavenger cells capable of engulfing and breaking down a wide variety of foreign substances.

Neutrophils—Cells, capable of phagocytosis, which are a major factor in acute inflammatory reactions.

Phagocytosis—The process in which macrophages and neutrophils take up foreign particles.

Plasma cells—Lymphoid cells, derived from B-cells, which produce antibodies.

Rejection—The process by which an individual's immune defenses destroy foreign cells or tissues.

Spleen—An organ in the abdominal cavity that can be an important site of antibody production, especially against antigens that invade the blood stream.

Thymus—An organ located in the forward part of the chest that is highly important to the immunological defense system, especially during childhood. In man the organ diminishes during adult life.

T-Cell—Also called a T-lymphocyte, key factor in cell mediated immunity. The cells are called T-cells because they are acted upon by the thymus to achieve their mature state.

Transfer factor—A soluble substance which can be harvested from the blood of humans. It will transfer to a nonimmune person in whom it is injected, certain kinds of immunity against antigens to which the donor was immune.

Vaccine—Originally the protective agent against smallpox. Now any material, containing antigens of a disease-causing germ, which will stimulate active immunity to that germ in the person who receives the vaccination.

White cells—General term for leukocytes and lymphocytes.

SUGGESTED
FURTHER READING

The scientific literature of immunology is vast. For those who wish to go deeper into this and related subjects, the following are suggested as an introduction:

Report of the Task Force on Immunology and Disease of the National Institute of Allergy and Infectious Diseases, 1973.

Report of the Fourth International Congress of the Transplantation Society, Transplantation, 1973.

Genetic Control of Immune Responsiveness, Hugh O. McDevitt and Maurice Landy, editors (New York: Academic Press, 1972).

Immunologic Intervention, Jonathan W. Uhr and Maurice Landy, editors (New York: Academic Press, 1971).

Immune Surveillance, Richard T. Smith and Maurice Landy, editors (New York: Academic Press, 1970).

Mediators of Cellular Immunity, H. Sherwood Lawrence and Maurice Landy, editors (New York: Academic Press, 1969).

Immunological Tolerance, Maurice Landy and Werner Braun, editors (New York: Academic Press, 1969).

Immunoglobulins, Annals of the New York Academy of Sciences, Vol. 190, Editors Shaul Kochwa and Henry G. Kunkel, 1971.

Immunology and Disease, The report of a Task Force on Immunology and Disease, National Institute of Allergy and Infectious Diseases, National Institutes of Health, (Washington: U.S. Government Printing Office, In Press).

A Second Look at Life, Felix T. Rapaport, editor (New York: Grune & Stratton, 1973).

Rh, The Intimate History of a Disease and its Conquest, David R. Zimmerman (New York: Macmillan Publishing Company, Inc., 1973).

Progress in Immunology, Proceedings of the First International Congress of Immunology, D. Bernard Amos, editor (New York: Academic Press, 1971).

Immunobiology, Robert A. Good and David W. Fisher, editors (Stamford, Conn: Sinauer Associates, Inc., 1971).

Immunologic Deficiency Diseases in Man. Birth Defects, Original Articles Series, Vol. IV, No. 1, February, 1968 (New York: The National Foundation).

The Semi-Artificial Man, Harold M. Schmeck, Jr. (New York: Walker and Company, 1965).

Slow, Latent and Temperate Virus Infections, NINDB Monograph No. 2, D. Carleton Gajdusek, Clarence J. Gibbs, Jr., Michael Alpers, editors, Public Health Service Publication No. 1378 (Washington: U.S. Government Printing Office, 1965).

An ABS of Modern Immunology, E. J. Holboro (Boston: Little Brown and Company, 1968).

INDEX